D0732675

Acing the
GI Board Exam

THE ULTIMATE CRUNCH-TIME RESOURCE

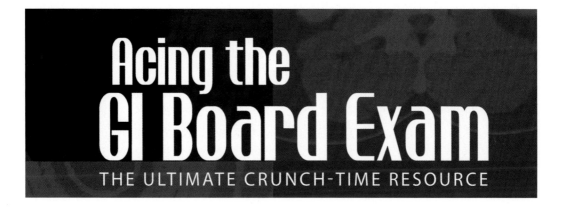

Acing the GI Board Exam

THE ULTIMATE CRUNCH-TIME RESOURCE

BRENNAN SPIEGEL, MD, MSHS

*Chief of Education and Training, UCLA
Division of Digestive Diseases*

*Director, UCLA/VA
Center for Outcomes Research and Education (CORE)*

*Assistant Professor of Medicine,
David Geffen School of Medicine at UCLA*

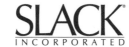

SLACK®
INCORPORATED

Delivering the best in health care information and education worldwide

www.slackbooks.com

ISBN: 978-1-55642-868-5

Copyright © 2009 by SLACK Incorporated

The procedures and practices described in this book should be implemented in a manner consistent with the professional standards set for the circumstances that apply in each specific situation. Every effort has been made to confirm the accuracy of the information presented and to correctly relate generally accepted practices. The authors, editor, and publisher cannot accept responsibility for errors or exclusions or for the outcome of the material presented herein. There is no expressed or implied warranty of this book or information imparted by it. Care has been taken to ensure that drug selection and dosages are in accordance with currently accepted/recommended practice. Due to continuing research, changes in government policy and regulations, and various effects of drug reactions and interactions, it is recommended that the reader carefully review all materials and literature provided for each drug, especially those that are new or not frequently used. Any review or mention of specific companies or products is not intended as an endorsement by the author or publisher.

SLACK Incorporated uses a review process to evaluate submitted material. Prior to publication, educators or clinicians provide important feedback on the content that we publish. We welcome feedback on this work.

Published by: SLACK Incorporated
                  6900 Grove Road
                  Thorofare, NJ 08086 USA
                  Telephone: 856-848-1000
                  Fax: 856-848-6091
                  www.slackbooks.com

Contact SLACK Incorporated for more information about other books in this field or about the availability of our books from distributors outside the United States.

Library of Congress Cataloging-in-Publication Data

Spiegel, Brennan M.R.
  Acing the GI board exam : the ultimate crunch-time resource / Brennan M.R. Spiegel.
  p. ; cm.
  Includes bibliographical references and index.
  ISBN 978-1-55642-868-5
  1. Gastroenterology--Case studies. 2. Gastroenterology--Examinations, questions, etc. 3. Gastroenterologists--Licenses--United States--Examinations--Study guides. I. Title.
  [DNLM: 1. Gastrointestinal Diseases--Examination Questions. WI 18.2 S755a 2009]
  RC808.S65 2009
  616.3'3--dc22
                          2009005694

Printed in the United States of America.

Last digit is print number: 10   9   8   7   6   5   4

DEDICATION

To my wife, Tracy, and children, Kaelen and Shane. Without them I'd be lost and confused. With them I am whole and sustained.

CONTENTS

ACKNOWLEDGMENTS

This book was greatly enhanced by the feedback and input from current and former GI fellows at UCLA. I am especially grateful to Benjamin Weinberg, who helped develop the title and who reviewed an initial draft of the manuscript. I'd also like to acknowledge Eric Esrailian and Hetal Karsan, who provided important feedback. I'd also like to thank Fred Weinstein, Binh Pham, and James Farrell for providing photographs for this book. And special thanks to Carrie Kotlar for her advocacy of the book, and to Debra Steckel for skillfully editing the manuscript. Finally, I must especially thank Fred Weinstein, my predecessor as GI Fellowship Director at UCLA, who allowed me to teach "Board review" to our fellows, despite his valid insistence that "Board review" is a concept that has little place in an academic University-based program. His stance has colored my own approach to this area, and helped me to remember that, after all, we're taking care of patients—not just trying to ace an exam.

ABOUT THE AUTHOR

Dr. Spiegel is Assistant Professor of Medicine in the Division of Digestive Diseases, UCLA School of Medicine, and in the Division of Gastroenterology, VA Greater Los Angeles Health Care System. He is the section chief for Health Services Research at the UCLA Division of Digestive Diseases, and Chief of Education and Training in the UCLA GI Fellowship Training Program—amongst the largest GI Training Programs in the country.

Dr. Spiegel attended Tufts University where he majored in Philosophy and Community Health, and obtained his medical degree from New York Medical College. He received training in internal medicine at Cedars-Sinai Medical Center in Los Angeles, completed a fellowship in Gastroenterology at UCLA, and completed advanced studies in Health Services Research in the UCLA School of Public Health, where he received a master's degree in Health Services. He is board certified in Internal Medicine and Gastroenterology. He currently teaches in the Schools of Medicine and Public Health at UCLA.

Dr. Spiegel's research interests have focused on acid-peptic disorders, chronic liver disease, gastrointestinal hemorrhage, and functional bowel disorders such as irritable bowel syndrome and dyspepsia. He has performed research across a range of health services methodologies, including health related quality of life measurement, survey design and administration, systematic review, meta-analysis, multivariable regression analysis, survival analysis, expert panel research, quality improvement, cost-effectiveness analysis, budget impact modeling, and use of clinical informatics to support decision making. He is a peer reviewer for numerous medical journals, and is on the editorial boards for the *American Journal of Gastroenterology* and *Clinical Gastroenterology and Hepatology*. He has contributed to the publication of more than 60 peer-reviewed papers, as well as numerous abstracts, book chapters, and monographs.

PREFACE

At this point in your career you know a lot. It's been a hard-earned battle, but after years of reading books, sitting through lectures, and working with patients, you now have a pretty good sense of what is important and what is, well, less important. You're also busy, and your time is limited. So now that you have to study for Boards or prepare for a clerkship, your goal is to learn the stuff you don't know, not review the stuff you already do know.

Yet, for some reason, we all continue to practice an inefficient approach to studying for Board exams. This usually consists of comprehensively reviewing the entirety of a topic area without thinking about: (a) whether we are adding incremental information to our preexisting storehouse of knowledge, and (b) whether we are learning things that are actually on the examination. Presumably you've already done the painstaking work of learning the basics of your trade. Now you have to get down to business and ace a test. Those are two very different activities.

Yet the inefficient approach to Board review is perennially fostered by traditional board review textbooks, in which content areas are laid out in chapter-by-chapter (and verse) detail, fully laden with facts both high and low yield—both relevant and irrelevant to actual examinations. There is a time and place for the chapter and verse approach to learning your trade, but Board review crunch time probably is not it. Yet, when I look back at my own efforts to study for Boards, I see page markings like this:

Chapter 1 – The Esophagus   **12**

Dysphagia is difficulty swallowing. There are two types of dysphagia: (a) transfer dysphagia, and (b) transit dysphagia. Transfer dysphagia is marked by an inability to transfer food from the oropharynx into the esophagus. Transit dysphagia is the inability to propel food down the esophagus into the stomach. Transit dyaphagia, in turn, may occur from both structural and functional abnormalities. Structural abnormalities include tumors, Zenker's diverticula, or strictures. Functional abnormalities include diffuse esophageal spasm, nutcracker esophagus, or aperistalsis. Achalasia is an example of both a structural and functional abnormality, as it is marked by: (1) hypertonic and thus obstructive lower esophageal sphincter (LES); (2) inability of the LES to relax with swallowing; and (3) esophageal aperistalsis.

I mean, you've got to be kidding! At the time I read that passage, I had already known that stuff since practically being in the womb—or, at least, since second year of medical school. Yet there is something self-gratifying about re-reading information that we already know and re-conquering content with a barrage of self-affirming scribbles, circles, stars, and highlights. Don't get me wrong: I have no problem with highlighting textbooks. I'm just saying that if you're going to spend time with a highlighter in Board review crunch time, you're better off spilling ink on stuff you never knew in the first place or had long forgotten, not on stuff that's already well ingrained.

But Board review books usually go a step further. They often present information that is actually not on the Boards (nor will ever be on the Boards), but that is merely of personal interest to the chapter authors. That is, many Board review books suffer from the affliction of academia running roughshod over practical information. This stuff is usually prefaced by the standard forerunners, like "Recent data indicate that...", or "Our group recently discovered that...", or "Although there is still a lack of consensus that...", and so forth. This kind of information is interesting and important for so many reasons, but it is not for Board review. When you're in crunch time, you shouldn't have to read about pet theories, areas of utter controversy (and thus ineligible for Board exams), or brand new or incompletely tested data that is too immature for Board exams. You need to know about time-tested pearls that show up year after year—not cutting edge hypotheses, novel speculations, new epidemiological oddities, or anything else not yet ready for "prime time." Board exams are about prime time.

This book is different. It aims for the "sweet spot" between what you already know, and what you don't already know (or forgot)—but that may be on the Boards. It tries to avoid the lower extreme of stuff you've known since birth, and the upper extreme of academic ruminations that are great for journal club or staying on the cutting edge, but that sit on the cutting room floor in Board exam editorial offices. You may find that you do know some of the stuff in this book and, if so, that's great. That means you're almost ready for the exam. But you'll also find that you don't know (or have forgotten) much of this book. And that is the point—you should be reading stuff you don't know, not reviewing content you already know well.

The information in this book has been culled from years of teaching "Board review" to our Gastroenterology ("GI") fellows at UCLA. I've come to realize that our fellows, who are amongst the best of the best, know a lot about their specialty, but are not necessarily ready for Boards. That's because we purposefully do not "teach for Boards" during everyday training—we instead teach the skills and knowledge that support rational and evidence-based decision-making in clinical practice. Unfortunately, Board exams don't always tap directly into those skill sets. Great clinicians can do poorly on Board exams. And great test takers can be suboptimal clinicians. We all recognize that it is primarily important to be a great clinician, and secondarily important to be a great test taker.

But with that caveat, it is still important to ace the Boards. And acing the Boards means that you ace not only the stuff you know, but also the "tough stuff" you may not yet know. And this tough stuff tends to recur year after year.

This book consists of a series of high yield vignettes on topics that are perennial Board review favorites, generally on the more difficult side, and full of pearls that may come in handy come Board time. All of these are originals—none is from an actual Board exam, naturally. But all have been endorsed, through an ongoing annual process of content development with our UCLA fellows, as being generally reflective of the kind of stuff that should show up on GI Board exams. It goes without saying that I have no idea what will be on your particular Board exam—and even if I did, I'm sure as heck not going to give you the answers in a book! Instead, I can make the more general statement that the stuff in this book is probably in the ballpark of things you should just know to help you on the exam.

Here are some highlights of this book:

- **Focus on clinical vignettes.** We see actual patients in clinical practice. And, to the Board's credit, most Board questions are clinical vignettes. This book presents questions in the form of clinical vignettes, not sterile, fact-laden blocks of text.

- **Relatively short.** Most Board review books are better suited for arm-curls than for rapidly and effectively teaching their content. Said another way, they are not "bathroom reading." Instead, most Board review books are read at a desk with a highlighter in hand. Unlike traditional didactic volumes, this book is big-time bathroom reading. You know, you sit down, open it up, and take in high-yield tough stuff in a hopefully entertaining format in short order. This is not a definitive text for comprehensive Board review, but a one-stop shop for high-impact stuff presented in a novel and interactive way. This book can be used in concert with longer volumes if you're looking for more extensive topic coverage.

- **Focus on stuff you don't know.** My reaction to reading usual Board review books: "I know this, I know this... Oh, that's interesting. "I know this, I know this... Oh, who knew? I know this, I know this, I know this... I'm bored." The goal of this book is for you to learn new stuff on every page, not to rehash stuff you already know. This book is relatively short—but it is dense with material you may not know yet. That's the point—learn stuff you don't know yet, don't keep reading and re-reading stuff you've known forever.

- **Emphasis on pearl after pearl after pearl.** Students, residents, fellows, and even attendings love clinical pearls. And so do the Boards. After every vignette in this book there is a pearl explicitly stated at the bottom called "Here's the Point..."

- **Random order of vignettes.** The Boards present questions in random order, not in nice, neat chapters. This book is meant to emulate the Board experience by providing vignettes in random order. It is a way to introduce cognitive dissonance into your learning by constantly switching directions. After all, patients appear in random order, so why not Board review material? If there is a specific topic you want to review, then you can check out the index and find the relevant pages. But again, keep in mind that this is not meant to be a treatise on any single topic, but instead a rapid-fire review of high-yield content.

- **No multiple-choice questions.** Multiple-choice questions are boring. They often test process of elimination more than knowledge and aptitude. When I teach Board review, I present a vignette, and then ask: "So what next?" Or: "What treatment will you give?" It's more entertaining. And it's more realistic. When patients come into an office, they don't have a multiple choice grid floating over their head in a hologram. So I find open-ended questions to be more engaging and interesting, even if the Boards emphasize multiple choice. Believe me—if you can get these questions right without multiple choice, then you'll most definitely get them right with multiple choice. There are other sources for straight-up multiple-choice question banks, such as those published by the American Board of Internal Medicine (ABIM).

- **Content reflective of ABIM proportions.** The ABIM writes and publishes the GI Board examination. The ABIM states that their exam content reflects an explicit percentage breakdown, as shown in Table 1. I have tried to maintain this proportion in the vignettes presented in this book. For a complete blueprint of the exam, as published by the ABIM, refer to: http://www.abim.org/pdf/blueprint/gastro_cert.pdf.

Table 1

OFFICIAL AMERICAN BOARD OF INTERNAL MEDICINE (ABIM) BREAKDOWN OF CONTENT AREAS ON THE GI BOARD EXAMINATION

Primary Content Areas	Relative Percentage of Examination
Liver	25%
Colon	15%
Stomach and Duodenum	15%
Esophagus	10%
Pancreas	10%
Small Intestine	10%
Biliary tract	8%
General (systemic disorders, nutrition, literature interpretation, statistics, epidemiology, ethics)	7%

- **Emphasis on "Clinical Thresholds."** I made up this idea of a "clinical threshold" after years of teaching Board review. The idea is that there are many Board-type questions that require the test taker to memorize some numerical threshold value. Like: "If the stool anion gap is less than XX, it's secretory diarrhea." Or: "If a subepithelial gastric mass is larger than Y cm, it must come out." And so forth. I've got around 100 of these values, and they come up year after year after year on the Boards. These are emphasized through the vignettes, and are separately catalogued towards the end of the book (page 189). The catalogue is a one stop shop for all the little numerical facts that everyone forgets but everyone needs to know. I often refer to this list myself, even as an attending, because it's so easy to forget some of these critical threshold values. This concept has caught on with our fellows, and the list of thresholds is now circulated every year to all the new fellows coming on service in July. For the first time, the full list is now formally presented in this book.

- **Comprehensive yet parsimonious explanations.** Some books provide multiple-choice questions and only give the letter answer. For example, the ABIM GI questions only have a letter answer without an explanation. Other books only provide a little tiny explanation. Others provide a full explanation, but with information that is not relevant. This book tries to provide a comprehensive answer to a non-multiple choice question while keeping it succinct and emphasizing the key clinical pearls. In other words, it attempts to give enough information to understand how to answer the question correctly without overwhelming the reader with additional details. Board review is not about ruminating forever about personal areas of interest—it is about cutting to the chase and keeping information on target.

- **Avoidance of mind-numbing prose.** Too many review books are boring as heck. They take away my will to live. When I was studying for Boards, I once fell asleep on my textbook and woke up in a pool of drool smearing some arcane motility tracing on the page beneath. That is no fun. This book is purposefully written in a manner that acknowledges that studying for Boards can be painful. I've tried to include interesting vignettes, provide answers that draw from real life clinical experience, and avoid unnecessary jargon or excessive academic descriptions.

- **Emphasis on images.** Clinical medicine is a visual art. And GI, in particular, is a visual subspecialty. The Boards acknowledge this by including lots of questions with images. Many of the vignettes in this book are accompanied by a carefully selected image designed to "bring the content to life" and aid in understanding the key points of the case.

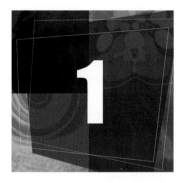

A COMPILATION OF GENERAL LESSONS LEARNED FROM TAKING THE GI BOARDS

General Observations

Over the years I have heard a lot of general impressions about the GI Board examination. Without any knowledge of specific content on the exam, here is a compilation of general lessons learned:

- **GI Boards are "Harder" than General Internal Medicine (GIM) Boards.** This is a virtually unanimous sentiment, and I had the same impression back when I took the exam. The GIM exam tends to emphasize breadth over depth. The challenge of preparing for the GIM exam is to know something about everything. In contrast, the challenge of preparing for the GI exam is to know a lot about fewer things—depth over breadth. As the saying goes: "Internists know less and less about more and more until they know nothing about everything. Specialists know more and more about less and less until they know everything about nothing." So your goal is to know "everything about nothing," so to speak. And knowing "everything" can be challenging, particularly when your time is limited. Most people who have taken both exams believe that knowing "everything about nothing" is generally harder than knowing "nothing about everything." These are obviously caricatures of reality—but there is also some truth to these caricatures.

- **GI Boards Demand Attention to Detail.** Because the GI exam (like other subspecialty exams) emphasizes depth over breadth, you really need to master the details of the content. General concepts and gestalt only go so far—at some point you need to have the details packed away in order to succeed on this test. And the test will probably push you to the limit on some of these details. For example, a classic clinical threshold is that a carcinoid >2 cm in the appendix requires right hemicolectomy, whereas a smaller lesion can be handled with a mere appendectomy. That is just a straight-up fact—1 of 100 listed in the Clinical Threshold Catalog on page 189. On the Boards, they might ask you how to handle a 1.8 cm lesion—not a 4 cm or 1 cm lesion, but a 1.8 cm lesion. In other words, they may go out of their way to find out if you really know the details, not "kind of" know the details. They'll push you right to the limit of the Clinical Threshold value. So you have to be prepared for this level of scrutiny. The GIM exam does not typically require that level of mastery.

- **GI Boards Highlight Minutiae.** In the Preface I mentioned that we do not typically teach for Boards. We teach what we see in real time, and, on average, we see "average stuff" in real time. But there is a bell-shaped curve of clinical content. The Board exam may push you to the extremes of that curve. It will probably require that you know all about conditions you may have never even seen (or only seen rarely)—like Hereditary Angioedema, Cronkhite-Canada Syndrome, cholesterol emboli to the colon, Tylosis, Blue Rubber Bleb Nevus Syndrome, Cowden's Syndrome, or Pseudoxanthoma Elasticum, among many other classics. And why shouldn't they ask about this stuff? If you don't know this material, then nobody will know this material, and the information will be lost forever in the textbooks. One purpose of Board review (and Board exams) is to ensure that you know not only the average run-of-the-mill stuff, but also the oddities that, over time, are sure to arrive in your office or clinic. And when they do arrive, chance will favor the prepared mind. So the Board exam wants to ensure that your mind is prepared, and that, should you ever see these entities, you will be equipped to recognize and treat them on a timely basis. You can call it "unfair" or "ridiculous" (terms I have heard before) that the exam always highlights these seemingly arcane topics. But, if you think about it, it is totally legitimate to test you on these conditions, even if they are widely considered to be "minutiae." The exam may also ask about seeming minutiae for common conditions. Rather than asking about the significance of a positive hydrogen lactulose breath test, the exam might ask about the significance of having megaloblastic anemia in the setting of a low B12 and high folate level. Both may be indicative of small intestinal bacterial overgrowth, but the latter is subtler than the former, and thus potentially more eligible to show up on an examination. Everyone knows that hydrogen breath tests are used to diagnose bacterial overgrowth. Not everyone knows that bacteria consume B12 and produce folate, and thus can yield the unusual pattern of a cobalamine-deficient megaloblastic anemia.

- **GI Boards Generally Assume You Already Know the Basics.** Every year I hear test takers complain that the exam did not ask any questions about the "common stuff." Of course, the exam undoubtedly did ask about common stuff, but probably did not ask about conditions in proportion to their actual clinical prevalence. For example, the year I took the exam, I remember leaving the test center thinking that there were virtually no questions on irritable bowel syndrome (IBS)—a condition that affects 10% to 20% of the population. But I seem to remember there being like 30 questions on Whipple's Disease. I also remembered that there were very few questions about the basic management of GI hemorrhage—stuff I had been doing through most of my call nights as a fellow. This theme seems to repeat itself every year. It leads me to believe that the Board examiners assume you already know the basics about everyday GI practice—ie, basic IBS management, basic endotherapy for GI bleeding, etc. I assume they test on that basic information in small quantities, from what I gather, but also want to ensure you know more than the basics. An internist knows the basics about GI. A GI needs to know just about everything about general GI.

Perennial Board Review "Favorites"

As mentioned in the preface, I have no idea what will show up on your exam. Moreover, I don't know anything about individual specific vignettes that have appeared on previous exams. I only know what we tend to emphasize in Board review, and topics we generally de-emphasize in Board review. Of course, this may or may not correspond with what shows up on your exam. With that caveat, here are some observations about general topics that tend to show up routinely:

- **Biliary Diseases and Endoscopic Retrograde Cholangiopancreatography (ERCP).** The official ABIM breakdown lists biliary disease as composing 8% of the examination. Pancreas makes up another 10%. So the combination means that nearly 1 in every 5 questions has something to do with pancreaticobiliary disorders. Many fellows do not spend a lot of time completing ERCPs or studying this branch of GI in much detail. I was one of those fellows. When I took the exam, I remember getting sideswiped by a battery of tough pancreaticobiliary questions. There were several cholangiograms, in particular, that had me scratching my head. At the time I just had not immersed myself sufficiently in the area, and I ended up paying for it. That was my lowest score of all the sections on the exam. So, it is important to familiarize yourself with all the basic cholangiograms, ie, annular pancreas; pancreas divisum; pancreaticopleural fistulae; "double duct" sign of pancreatic head cancer; type I, II, and III choledochal cysts; "string of lakes" of sclerosing cholangitis; Mirrizi's Syndrome; and so forth. They also seem to love pancreatitis. Another favorite is gallbladder polyps—a common condition that, for some reason, is rarely covered formally in typical GI Fellowship curricula. Pancreatic cysts may come up, but their management is often controversial, so don't expect detailed questions on how to manage, say, a 2-cm intraductal papillary mucinous neoplasm (IPMN). But you should be able to recognize the pathognomonic gelatinous ampullary ooze of IPMNs, know what to do with a symptomatic 3-cm IPMN, or know the basic management steps of a pancreatic pseudocyst, for example. Finally, acalculous cholecystitis is a Board review favorite, so it may pop up from time to time.

- **Pregnancy.** The Boards do love pregnancy. Pregnancy and inflammatory bowel disease, pregnancy and liver disease, pregnancy and GERD, pregnancy and [insert disease here]. You can't blame the Board for wanting to make sure you know this stuff—it is obviously critical. The problem is that most of you came to GI through internal medicine, and general internal medicine residencies are notorious for de-emphasizing pregnancy-related health and disease. It is no different in GI Fellowship training. When was the last time you did a full pelvic examination in a woman complaining of lower abdominal pain? Most GIs just don't do it routinely (for good or for bad—this is just an observation, not a judgment). In any event, the Board probably wants to make sure you know the basics about pregnancy. Classic Board review topics include: Acute Fatty Liver of Pregnancy (AFLP); Hemolysis, Elevated Liver enzymes, Low Platelets syndrome (HELLP); use of steroids in pregnancy; pregnancy classes of common GI medications (eg, PPIs); hyperemesis gravidarum, etc.

- **GI and Hepatic Manifestations of AIDS.** As with the GIM examination, AIDS and HIV-related illnesses will almost certainly be on the GI examination. It is important to know both luminal and hepatic manifestations of AIDS. High-yield Board review topics include: cryptosporidiosis, cytomegalovirus (CMV) anywhere in the GI tract, Kaposi's Sarcoma, HSV esophagitis, AIDS-related GI malignancies, *Mycobacterium avium* complex (MAC), reasons for fluconazole failure in esophageal candidiasis, and so forth. That list could go on for pages.

- **Polyps of All Types.** Polyps, polyps, polyps. If you can think of a polyp in the GI tract, there is a reasonable chance the exam will ask about it. Some Board review favorites include fibrovascular polyps of the esophagus, fundic gland polyps in the stomach, and duodenal polyps in familial adenomatous polyposis (FAP) and hereditary nonpolyposis colorectal cancer (HNPCC), among others.

- **Anything That Involves the Terminal Ileum (TI).** There always seems to be something about the TI. Know the extended differential diagnosis of terminal ileitis: eg, Crohn's Disease, backwash ileitis, tuberculosis, Yersinia, typhoid fever, cryptosporidiosis, radiation enteritis, actinomycosis, etc.

- **Nutritional Deficiencies.** The ABIM states that nutritional deficiencies compose a small part of the "general" category that makes up 7% of the exam. Thus, you might expect only 1 or 2 questions about nutritional deficiencies. So it is not necessarily high-yield to learn all the deficiencies from the standpoint of total questions, but it is high-yield from the standpoint of likelihood to show up on the exam, even if in small numbers. Perennial Board review favorites include zinc deficiency, biotin deficiency, and selenium deficiency (cardiomyopathy), among others. If you are in crunch time, it is almost a sure bet that spending 20 minutes on the deficiencies will yield at least a couple of correct answers.

- **Basic Epidemiology.** As with nutritional deficiencies, epidemiology is stowed away in the "general" category, and you can once again expect a handful (at most) of questions covering basic epidemiological principles. This is also the case for the GIM exams, along with nearly every other ABIM examination across specialties. Important topics include: difference between lead time and length time bias, sensitivity vs specificity, positive vs negative predictive value, definition of a P-value, and definition of 95% confidence intervals, among others. Bottom line with these: if you don't know these by now, it might be hard to learn them on short notice, and maybe you are better off focusing on other high-yield content. But as an evidence-based medicine maven myself, I encourage you to know this stuff—if for no other reason than you are virtually guaranteed to see some of this show up on the exam, since there are only so many permutations on this theme to work with.

- **Dermatological Manifestations of GI/Hepatic Diseases.** This is a favorite Board review topic because it reminds all of us that we are internists first, and sub-specialists second. Moreover, it is just easy to test this stuff because the content is a set-up for picture images. It is a high-yield activity to review images for all the major GI-dermatology links, including acanthosis nigricans with visceral malignancy, erythema nodosum with IBD (and others), pyoderma gangrenosum with IBD, the "sign of Lesser Trelat" with colon cancer, Blue Rubber Bleb Nevus Syndrome, "plucked chicken skin" in pseudoxanthoma elasticum, lip lesions in Osler Webber Rendu and Peutz-Jegher's Syndrome, acrodermatitis in zinc deficiency, dermatitis herpetiformis in celiac sprue, keratoderma in tylosis, trichilemmomas in Cowden's Syndrome, fissured tongue in Melkersson-Rosenthal Syndrome, and migratory necrolytic erythema in glucagonoma, among many others.

- **Hereditary Colorectal Cancer Syndromes.** This is an important topic for so many reasons, not the least of which is its likely appearance on Board exams. This topic is vulnerable ground, because many Fellows never really learn the details about common hereditary syndromes, including HNPCC (and the Muir-Torre variant of HNPCC in particular), FAP, Peutz-Jegher's Syndrome, Cowden's Syndrome, Tuberous Sclerosis, and Juvenile Polyposis, among others. I have ensured that this book includes vignettes on each of these common topics.

- **Metabolic Liver Diseases.** It is almost a guarantee that you will be asked about Wilson's Disease, Hereditary Hemochromatosis (HHC), or α-1 antitrypsin (AT) deficiency. Just know these. Classic Board review "factlets" include: treat HCV before HHC in HCV-infected patients, low ALP is seen in Wilson's Disease, PAS+ globules accumulated in hepatocytes is seen in α-1 AT, and so forth.

- **Hepatitis C Virus (HCV) Infection.** This is 1 example where the prevalence of the disease in the community should be matched by its prevalence on the examination itself. The general feedback has been that HCV questions are relatively common, but also relatively "easy" compared to other areas of the examination. As with Hepatitis B, HCV remains a rapidly changing area, so you will generally be held accountable for older, well-supported facts, not recent innovations or cutting-edge data from the newest combination therapies.

Generally De-Emphasized Topics

In contrast to the topics outlined above, there are other areas of GI that have been historically de-emphasized in Board review. Of course, that does not mean that next year's exam won't be filled to the brim with these topics. And furthermore, "generally de-emphasized" does not mean absent from the exam altogether—just de-emphasized compared to other topics. In any event, these areas probably get relatively short shrift on the exam:

- **Functional GI Disorders.** Functional GI disorders (FGID), such as IBS, chronic idiopathic constipation, functional dyspepsia, and functional abdominal pain syndrome (among many others) are extremely common in everyday clinical practice. They are the bane of our outpatient existence. Yet despite their overwhelming clinical prevalence, their prevalence on the Boards will probably be mismatched, with relatively few questions covering this expansive area of GI. The seeming de-emphasis on FGIDs might occur for several reasons, including: (1) management remains uncertain for most of these disorders, making it difficult for examiners to create extensive question sets in the absence of clear-cut clinical management guidelines; (2) examiners may assume that test takers already know the basics for how to manage most FGIDs, and thus reserve their questions to target other conditions where knowledge may be less complete (although it can easily be argued that many graduating fellows have incomplete knowledge about FGIDs, thus the importance to test on this topic); or (3) there might not be many FGID mavens writing Board questions, and thus other areas of personal interest tend to crowd out the FGIDs despite their overwhelming clinical prevalence. Whatever the explanation, there have historically been few "tough" questions about IBS, functional dyspepsia, constipation, and so forth. Maybe this will change in time. I suspect that as long as experts are confused about how best to manage these disorders, examiners will continue to de-emphasize FGIDs when writing questions, and instead focus on conditions where the disease paradigm and management approaches are more streamlined and standardized.

- **Motility Tracings.** I wouldn't be surprised if there were a couple of motility tracings on the Board exam, but these probably won't go beyond the basics. It is worth knowing some key motility patterns, including the Big Four: diffuse esophageal spasm, nutcracker esophagus, achalasia (and vigorous achalasia), and pelvic dyssynergia, in particular. Beyond those basics, it is unlikely that the Boards would present complicated motility tracings that require specialized knowledge to interpret. It is clear that most graduating fellows have not received extensive training in motility tracing interpretation, so it is not really "fair" to expect test takers to be able to interpret complex or mixed patterns of disease in the context of an exam. But, it is definitely high yield to know the Big Four patterns. Just don't spend too much time ruminating about variations beyond this core group. Your crunch time will probably be better spent doing other things once you have mastered the basics. The Big Four patterns are covered in this book.

- **pH Tracings and Impedence.** You should be able to distinguish pathological amounts of acid reflux from physiologic reflux. The "rule of 4s" should get you through most of these questions (pH<4 for >4% time). Impedence monitoring is a newer technology that has not been widely disseminated, but it is reasonable to expect that the examiners may soon (if not already) ask about how to interpret a simple impedence tracing. It is worth knowing about impedence if you don't already, because it is an interesting technology that is potentially clinically useful. But beyond the basics, you should not be called upon to interpret complex pH tracings or complicated impedence patterns. Similarly, it is unlikely that you will need to interpret varying combinations of reflux-to-symptom ratios, mostly because those metrics were primarily designed for research purposes and are not widely validated or clinically employed. Bottom line is that, like motility tracings, you probably should not dedicate too much time to learning complex pH or impedence patterns, and instead should focus on knowing the bare-bones basics in terms of tracing interpretation. That is not to say there won't be questions on GERD management in general—that is an expansive and important topic. But the specific area of pH and impedence tracings should be relatively de-emphasized. Maybe this will change in time.

- **GI Hemorrhage.** Similar to the FGIDs, GI hemorrhage is a common clinical problem that is not necessarily "common" on the Boards. I suspect that the exams probably are asking about GI hemorrhage, but that test takers just don't remember the topic arising because the questions were relatively straightforward. Test takers usually remember the "tough stuff," not the "gimmies." In any event, I suspect there are relatively few tough questions about GI bleed management, and that knowing the basics (eg, how to endoscopically handle different stigmata of recent hemorrhage, how to dose intravenous PPI therapy, optimal timing of endoscopy in high-risk bleeders, etc) from your training is probably sufficient to get you through most of those questions. If you have not been exposed to much GI bleeding during your fellowship, which would be unusual, then perhaps you'll want to ensure you know the basics and spend a bit more time reviewing this area. But if you have been actively performing hemostasis and managing inpatient GI bleeders, you are probably well on your way to correctly answering most of the relevant Board questions on this topic.

- **Device/Technology Issues.** We spend a lot of time in everyday clinical GI figuring out which scope to use, which catheter to float, which balloon to deploy, or whether to use clips vs bipolar probes, among other device topics. Device and technology issues are vital in GI. But the Boards are unlikely to ask much about these areas. For example, the examiners are probably more interested in knowing which general technique you will use when faced with achalasia-related dysphagia, not whether you will use a 30-mm vs 40-mm rigid balloon dilator. Similarly, the examiners will be more interested in making sure you do not apply endotherapy to a flat pigmented spot, not whether you are using a single vs double channel scope in a GI bleeder (although scope size is critical in GI bleeding—just not something typically covered in Board review). Again, it is certainly possible that the exam will start to delve into these technical topics in time, but, historically at least, this type of information has not been heavily emphasized.

- **Non-Biliary Radiology.** You do need to know basic cholangiograms, as previously discussed, but the Board examiners should hopefully recognize that you are a gastroenterologist—not a radiologist. Even though GI relies heavily on abdominal imaging in everyday clinical practice, it is expected that we are working with radiologists when interpreting images. So you should rarely, if ever, be given a radiograph without any supporting information. Typically there should be enough information in the vignette to piece together what is happening in the image, even if you can't actually interpret the image. It is still useful to recognize basic radiographic patterns (eg, ascites, bowel obstruction, "target-sign" of intussusception, liver masses, terminal ileal disease, bowel infarction, etc), but at this point you pretty much know what you know when it comes to GI imaging. It will be generally low-yield to spend Board review crunch time carefully studying different CT, MR, or ultrasound images. If you were going to carefully study images, I would recommend spending some time with cholangiograms instead. For non-biliary questions, you will have to rely on your general knowledge about imaging and couple that with your specific knowledge about GI, since the accompanying vignettes will have sufficient data to allow correct answers even if you can't precisely interpret the provided image.

- **Pathology Interpretation.** Pathology interpretation is a fundamental skill for practicing gastroenterologists. Every biopsy we take needs pathologic interpretation, and the results almost always have important clinical implications. But at the same time, we are gastroenterologists, not pathologists. Similar to the radiology discussion, it should be the case that Board questions tied to pathology results will also provide sufficient information to answer the question without having to precisely interpret the histopathology. Undoubtedly, you need to know some basic patterns of histopathology: intestinal metaplasia in Barrett's, interface hepatitis with plasma cells in autoimmune hepatitis, Marsh lesions in celiac sprue, foveolar hyperplasia in Menetrier's, PAS+ foamy macrophages in Whipple's and MAC, and cystic dilations of fundic gland polyps, among many other Board review favorites (see vignettes 137-149). But in each of these cases, the exam should provide concurrent clinical information, and you should be able to piece together the answer without being an expert in histopathological interpretation. In situations where you are called upon to directly interpret a pathology slide, chances are the abnormality will be right under your nose and "classic"—not some strange variation. Leave it to the pathologists to be experts in interpreting fine degrees of separation between conditions. You should know the basics, and be able to tie those basics to clinical information. I predict that the Boards will pull out the pathognomonic "classics" when it comes to requiring histopathologic interpretation.

- **Liver Transplantation.** Hepatology is an exploding field, and the GI Board exam does heavily emphasize this field. In fact, the ABIM states that 1 in 4 Board questions pertains to hepatology (see Table 1). So, if you are not a big "liver fan," now is the time to become one, because you have to know liver. But, there is a fine line between the hepatology that a general GI should know, and the specialized knowledge that a hepatologist should know. This is not a test for budding hepatologists. There is a move afoot to better define the hepatology curriculum, and to create a separate examination for this burgeoning field. Liver transplantation, in particular, is a very specialized area that is generally reserved for "official" hepatologists. It is not expected that community gastroenterologists know how to manage posttransplant patients, in particular. Pretransplant issues, such as staging with Model for End Stage Liver Disease (MELD), are relevant to practicing GIs and should be on the Board examination. But peri- and postoperative transplant topics should not be heavily emphasized on the general GI examination. If you are in crunch time, it is probably low-yield to start learning this stuff, particularly if you have not already been exposed to post-liver transplant patients in much detail. But know the basics: what is MELD? How is MELD used?

What are the indications and contraindications to liver transplant? What are the Milan criteria for liver masses and transplant eligibility?... and so forth. If you can answer these basic questions, then you should be well on your way to getting the basic transplant-related questions correct on the Boards.

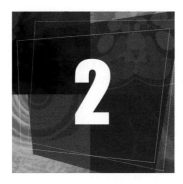

"TOUGH STUFF" VIGNETTES

In the pages that follow are 160 "tough stuff" vignettes. As described in the Preface, these have been culled from years of teaching Board review, and have been iteratively reviewed and vetted with our fellows at UCLA. As you go through these vignettes, keep the following points in mind:

- These are generally difficult. That is by design. You may nonetheless know the answers for many of these vignettes—a sign that you are well prepared for the exam. But if you can't get them all right, that is fine too. That is the whole point of this book—to ensure that you are gaining incremental information, not just reviewing stuff you already know. Keep in mind, however, that for every "tough" question that is in this book, there are a bunch of "gimmies" that do not appear in this book. The entire Board exam won't be full of "tough stuff" questions. So don't get too demoralized if you can't correctly answer all of these. Rest assured that you already know most of the "gimmies" just by virtue of paying attention and learning during your clinical experiences.

- These are in completely random order—there is no explicit rhyme or reason. Although the question set roughly complies with the ABIM percentage breakdown previously described in Table 1 of the Preface, these are purposefully not in any rational order. See the Preface for my rationale for this setup.

- The Vignettes appear on 1 page, followed by 1 or more open-ended questions. The answers are provided on the next page. Before you turn the page, take a moment to really think about the answers. Even if you are not sure of the answer, at least take a moment to think about the potential differential diagnosis, or other information you might need to better answer the question. This form of active learning is more useful than merely flipping the page and reading the answer.

- After each answer there is a short section entitled "Why might this be tested?" The purpose of this entry is to emphasize why it is important to know the content of each vignette, vis a vis the Board exam in particular. It puts you in the mind of the Board examiners for a second to better understand their potential reasoning, and might help you better remember each vignette.

- At the bottom of each answer page there is a box entitled: "Here's the Point!" This is meant to summarize the key issue or issues that appear on the page. If you are really in crunch time, then you should, at the very least, make sure you know the "Here's the Point" bottom line for each vignette. The Crunch-Time Self Test on page 197 catalogs all of these factlets (and more) into a 170 question test, and quizzes you to see if you can remember the key points from each vignette.

- Some of the answer pages also have a "Clinical Threshold Alert," followed by the presentation of an explicit clinical threshold (see the Preface for details). One hundred of these Clinical Thresholds are fully cataloged on page 189 for your convenience during crunch time.

Vignette 1: Elevated Liver Tests and Conjunctival Suffusion

A 52-year-old man is referred to you for evaluation of abnormal liver tests. The abnormalities developed in association with a multi-system illness that began 10 days after participating in a triathlon that included swimming in a natural lake. The patient was in his usual state of health until he developed progressive fevers, muscle tenderness, rigors, abdominal pain, diarrhea, and a nonproductive cough. He presented to his primary care provider who diagnosed a viral syndrome and prescribed 650 mg of acetaminophen 3 times daily as necessary. The symptoms persisted, and he then developed yellow eyes, progressive fatigue, and high fevers. He reported taking acetaminophen only intermittently, and never more than twice daily. He only drinks alcohol occasionally, takes occasional low-dose aspirin for cardioprophylaxis, and does not use any herbal remedies.

His vital signs are remarkable for a temperature of 101.9° and a heart rate of 59. On examination he is found to have prominent conjunctival suffusion, along with icterus. There are no stigmata of chronic liver disease. He has a large spleen and a smooth, nontender liver edge palpated 3 cm below the right costal margin. There are no ascites. He has palpable, nontender lymph nodes in his neck and groin bilaterally. His muscles are tender to palpation in his upper and lower extremities.

Relevant laboratories include: Total Bilirubin=8.9; AST=196; ALT=172; ALP=229; Albumin=3.8; INR=1.0; Hgb=13.2; Platelet=366; WBC=14.6 (81% PMNs); Sodium=129; Potassium=3.2; Bicarbonate=24; BUN=39; Creatinine=1.6; Creatinine Kinase=1000; acetaminophen level=undetectable; ethanol level=undetectable.

▶ **What is the diagnosis?**

▶ **What is the treatment?**

Vignette 1: Answer

This is Weil's Syndrome from infection with *Leptospira interrogans.* Weil's syndrome is a severe form of leptospirosis that can involve the liver. Leptospirosis is usually transmitted through urine from small rodents. There was a huge outbreak of this from a triathlon in Illinois in 2002—the inspiration for this vignette. In that instance, the outbreak was traced back to exposure to lake water that was probably contaminated with rodent-infected urine (lovely). Leptospirosis is one of those conditions that can do just about anything, and a full overview of the disease is beyond the scope of this brief review.

But you should know the classic characteristics, which include high fever with a temperature-pulse dissociation (as seen here), marked conjunctival suffusion, myalgias, fevers, nonproductive cough, lymphadenopathy, and rigors. When severe, it can lead to rhabdomyolysis, renal insufficiency, electrolyte abnormalities (hyponatremia and hypokalemia), and liver abnormalities. Fulminant liver failure is rare. Instead, the liver dysfunction is more of an epiphenomenon from the overall illness—not a central factor. Patients with Weil's syndrome typically have transaminases in the sub-200 range, and may have elevated bilirubin and ALP levels. In fact, the bilirubin has been reported to be as high as 60 to 80 mg/dL in some severe cases.

The diagnosis relies upon serological testing, either with a microscopic agglutination test, which is difficult to perform and not widely available, or a rapid serologic test with an IgM ELISA assay. Most cases of leptospirosis are self-limited and do not require antibiotics. Treatment is usually with doxycycline. The differential diagnosis is broad, but in this case nearly all of the classic findings are in place. Acetaminophen toxicity should always be kept in mind, but generally patients must ingest more than 7.5 g of acetaminophen (or 150 mg/kg) in order to precipitate liver failure. In this case the levels are undetectable. It would be reasonable to also check for viral hepatitis serologies, but viral hepatitis would not typically present with this overall symptom complex (eg, temperature-pulse dissociation, conjunctival suffusion, cough, renal insufficiency, all after a triathlon).

Why might this be tested? Because it is easy to miss this diagnosis. When we think about acute hepatitis, we don't usually think about Leptospirosis. Yet this infection is eminently treatable. Keep it on the radar, particularly if there is any sniff of possible rodent urine exposure (yikes), like fresh water swimming, barefoot in bathrooms with open foot sores (rare, but has been known to happen), etc.

Clinical Threshold Alert: If more than 7.5 g (or 150 mg/kg) of acetaminophen is consumed at once, then acetaminophen can be hepatotoxic.

Here's the Point!

Swimming in Lake (or equivalent) + Elevated Bilirubin + Conjunctival Suffusion + Temperature-Pulse Dissociation = Leptospirosis (Weil's Syndrome)

Vignette 2: Diarrhea, Heart Failure, and Neuropathy

A 59-year-old man with rheumatoid arthritis (RA) presents with chronic diarrhea. The symptoms first began 18 months ago and have been progressively worse over time. He describes his BMs as non-bloody, "flaky," and "like oatmeal." He reports early satiety and meal-related nausea and bloating. He has lost 20 pounds unintentionally over the last year.

Review of systems reveals lower extremity swelling, orthopnea, dyspnea on exertion, and fatigue. He complains of progressive abdominal swelling. In addition, he reports tingling in his bilateral hands and legs in a "stocking and glove" distribution.

On physical exam he is found to have orthostatic vital signs. There is an S3 gallop. His liver is enlarged, and there is evidence of ascites. There are no spider angiomata, no palmar erythema, and no asterixis. Neurological exam reveals evidence of peripheral sensory and motor neuropathy. Relevant laboratories include: AST=84; ALT=66; ALP=249; albumin=2.1; serum carotene=8.

▶ *What is the most likely diagnosis?*

▶ *How can you confirm the diagnosis?*

Vignette 2: Answer

This is secondary amyloidosis. Amyloidosis is one of those conditions that, should you fall asleep in morning report and be abruptly awakened to provide a potential diagnosis, you can propose this condition and everyone in the room will nod knowingly.

Basically, amyloidosis can do just about anything. In this case, the patient has RA, which is a tip-off for reactive or secondary amyloidosis. Recall that reactive amyloidosis is associated with so-called AA amyloid fibrils—an acute phase reactant—whereas primary amyloidosis is associated with AL amyloid fibrils, which are monoclonal light chains. Gastrointestinal involvement is most common in reactive amyloidosis, and typically involves several pathological mechanisms, including mucosal infiltration (leading to malabsorption), neuromuscular infiltration (leading to dysmotility and stasis), and extrinsic autonomic neuropathy (also leading to dysmotility and, in this patient, peripheral neuropathy and orthostatic hypotension).

This patient has symptoms suggestive of gastroparesis, which is common in reactive amyloidosis. The bloating suggests dysmotility and possible small intestinal bacterial overgrowth—also a consequence of dysmotility and stasis. The "oatmeal consistency" diarrhea indicates possible fat malabsorption, which is further confirmed by the low serum carotene levels. In addition, amyloid can infiltrate the liver. This typically presents with an enlarged liver, ascites, and an ALP elevated out of proportion to the transaminases, thus suggesting a diffuse infiltrative disease. It is notable that presence of hepatic amyloid is associated with a higher risk of hemorrhage from liver biopsy (see Vignette 39 for additional details). Amyloid can also deposit in the heart and lead to heart failure from a restrictive cardiomyopathy, which is also evidenced in this patient.

The diagnosis can be confirmed with either a fat pad biopsy or a rectal biopsy (latter is more sensitive). When performing the rectal biopsy, be sure to target vessels with the biopsy forceps, since amyloid is preferentially deposited in the blood vessels, as evidenced by the classic Congo Red angiopathy. Figure 2-1 presents microscopy of the classic changes. Although not evidenced in this case, amyloid can also lead to GI bleeding through vascular friability and formation of mucosal lesions. If primary amyloid is suspected, then you should also check for presence of a serum Bence Jones Protein. But even when present, you should still go a step further and biopsy either duodenal or rectal mucosa (latter is more accessible and thus generally preferred) to confirm the diagnosis.

The treatment of GI and hepatic amyloidosis is challenging and often ineffective. The first principle is to treat the underlying condition—in this case RA. Patients with bloating and diarrhea should be tested for bacterial overgrowth and treated if positive (or even if just suspected, regardless of the test results). Those with delayed gastric emptying should receive a prokinetic therapy as tolerated. Protein-losing enteropathy may be treated with corticosteroids or octreotide with variable success.

Why might this be tested? This is a classic diagnosis because it affects nearly every organ system, and is particularly troublesome for the GI tract. It also requires you to identify a wide range of GI and hepatology disorders, including gastroparesis, small intestinal bacterial overgrowth, protein-losing enteropathy, ascites, and infiltrative liver disease, among others.

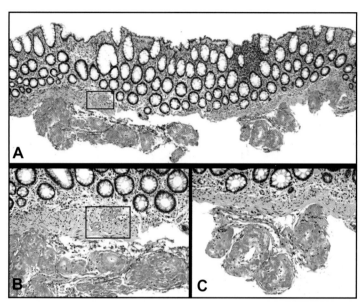

Figure 2-1. Amyloid Congo Red Stain. A) Low power shows large numbers of vessels in the submucosa positive-staining. Small amyloid deposits are commonly seen in the muscularis mucosae (Box) and B) Higher power. C) Dense deposits are clearly seen in the submucosal blood vessels. (Courtesy of Wilfred Weinstein, MD, David Geffen School of Medicine at UCLA.)

Here's the Point!

Diarrhea + Dysmotility + Heart Failure + Neuropathy = Amyloid

Vignette 3: Third Trimester Jaundice

A 26-year-old G1P0 woman is referred by her primary care physician for new-onset jaundice. She first noticed that her eyes were yellow during week 28 of pregnancy, and by week 30 she become "yellow all over." She now has nausea, recurrent diarrhea, diffuse muscle aches, and progressive fatigue. She has not been drinking alcohol during her pregnancy, and has no significant history of alcohol abuse prior to her pregnancy. She has no abdominal pain.

On examination she is alert, fully oriented, has no evidence of asterixis, and has normal deep tendon reflexes. She has icteric sclerae. Her abdomen is gravid and consistent with dates. It is difficult to palpate her liver, but there is no clear evidence of hepatomegaly. Her abdomen is non-tender. She has 2 spider angiomata on her anterior chest. She has no palmar erythema, no caput medusa, and no evidence of ascites.

Her laboratory values are notable for an AST of 452, ALT of 550, and a total bilirubin of 3.2. Her albumin=3.3, INR=1.1, platelets=140.

▶ *What is the most likely diagnosis?*

▶ *What cause of this diagnosis needs urgent treatment?*

Vignette 3: Answer

This is acute viral hepatitis. It is easy to get this wrong because it is almost too obvious. The usual temptation is to think about pregnancy-related conditions such as acute fatty liver of pregnancy (AFLP) and HELLP syndrome. AFLP is incorrect because it tends to occur later in pregnancy (late third trimester), is variably associated with low glucose, elevated creatinine, elevated international normal ratio (INR), a higher total bilirubin, and low-normal platelets, and is generally much less common than run-of-the-mill viral hepatitis. HELLP is unlikely because it also tends to occur later in pregnancy (although it can occur as early as the late second trimester), is more common in multiparous women, is variably associated with an elevated creatinine, and is marked by a lower platelet count.

The point here is that acute viral hepatitis is common, and pregnant women are equally eligible to get viral hepatitis as non-pregnant women (or men, for that matter). Whereas non-HSV, non-Hepatitis E viral hepatitis rarely affects pregnancy adversely, HSV hepatitis in particular may be fatal in up to 50% of cases. This entity mandates urgent treatment with an appropriate agent, such as acyclovir or vidarabine. Assuming this entity has been excluded, treatment usually consists of supportive therapy. Also, do not forget that spider angiomata are normal in pregnancy, particularly if there are only 2 or 3 identified.

Why might this be tested? Because the Board reviewers always have questions on pregnant women, and particularly like questions about pregnant women with third-trimester jaundice. Also, this is a simple test to see if you are over thinking the obvious and can prioritize the pre-test likelihood of various diseases in a differential diagnosis.

Here's the Point!

In a yellow pregnant woman, think about viral hepatitis if the question asks for the "most likely" diagnosis, regardless of the trimester.

Vignette 4: The "Snapping Uvula"

A 34-year-old man presents with a 6-month history of a "snapping uvula." He says that he intermittently coughs up a long, tubular piece of tissue that "snaps" out of his mouth, and then, as quickly as it emerged, "snaps back into the throat." His primary care physician told him the lesion was probably just a "long uvula," and not to worry. But he also has developed a sense of "fullness" in his throat, and thinks he occasionally has difficulty swallowing thick pieces of chicken or steak, although he has no dysphagia to liquids. He has no weight loss, no hematemesis, no melena, and no chest or abdominal pain. He reports no significant constitutional symptoms.

On a recent date night he choked on a piece of steak and vomited at the table. His girlfriend was amazed and frightened to see a fleshy tube snap out of his mouth and then snap back in. She ran away in horror. Now he is questioning the diagnosis of a long uvula, and has come to you for some advice. He also hopes you can help him get his girlfriend back with some rational explanation for whatever is going on!

▶ ***What the heck is this?***

▶ ***What can be done about it?***

Vignette 4: Answer

This is a fibrovascular polyp of the esophagus. I have seen a couple of these cases, but they are generally uncommon—a perfect setup for a Board question. Although it may be tempting to blame this bizarre set of symptoms on a large uvula, it would take a very large uvula to lead to a globus sensation, dysphagia, and a lesion that comes out beyond the incisors with vomiting.

This sounds more like an elongated polyp, which is exactly what it is. Fibrovascular polyps are benign growths that are almost exclusively situated at the upper esophageal sphincter near the cricoid. For whatever reason, they are reported more commonly in males—another tip off from the vignette.

The reason they are important to know, besides making for amazing stories, is that they can lead to asphyxiation when they are long. That is the real point here—they can be life threatening, not just date threatening! Many experts suggest performing endoscopic ultrasound (EUS) of the lesion once identified. This can establish whether there are any large penetrating vessels, which is important given the vascular nature of these lesions. If there is a large vessel, then snare polypectomy can be risky, and surgical cure is warranted.

If the lesion is <2 cm and lacks penetrating vessels, then snare polypectomy can be attempted. If the lesion is >2 cm then surgery is often performed regardless of whether there are penetrating vessels.

Why might this be tested? Because it is just totally crazy. But also, because if you fail to recognize this entity, then patients can asphyxiate and die. The Boards always want to make sure you can identify the dangerous stuff, and this seemingly benign condition can indeed be dangerous.

Here's the Point!

Weird Oral Projection + Globus + Dysphagia = Fibrovascular Polyp

Vignette 5: Colonic Nodules and Anemia

A 78-year-old woman is referred for microcytic, iron-deficiency anemia. This was first detected after she developed progressive fatigue and was evaluated by her primary care physician.

Laboratories revealed the following: Hgb=9.8; MCV=78; Ferritin=18; Iron Saturation=30%. In addition to iron deficiency anemia, concurrent labs revealed an ESR of 86, and a WBC of 8.2 with 80% eosinophils.

She has a history of ischemic heart disease, renovascular disease, and repair of an abdominal aortic aneurysm. Her physical examination is notable for bruits over her carotid and femoral arteries. You perform an upper endoscopy that is normal. Colonoscopy reveals multiple small, raised, focal nodules in the sigmoid and transverse colon. Biopsy results subsequently reveal intra-arteriolar needle-shaped clefts within the specimens.

▶ **What is the diagnosis?**

Vignette 5: Answer

This is cholesterol embolization to the GI tract. It turns out that the GI tract is the third most common site of cholesterol embolization. Characteristic features of cholesterol embolization, in general, include an elevated ESR and eosinophilia. The history of cardiovascular comorbidities and advanced atherosclerosis, in particular, are risk factors for this entity. GI involvement may present with abdominal pain, diarrhea, and GI bleeding.

The characteristic mucosal lesion is a yellowish, raised nodule, which may occur throughout the GI tract. On mucosal biopsy there are needle-shaped clefts (Board buzzword) which correspond with the "negative image" of the previous cholesterol crystals, now gone from the specimen but leaving behind their footprints. Treatment includes standard management of hypercholesterolemia, including statins, risk factor management (smoking, diabetes), and minimizing the use of intravascular procedures where possible.

Why might this be tested? Because it is a marriage of general internal medicine and GI, and because there are so many "test-worthy" characteristics of this entity (high ESR, high eosinophils, needle-shaped clefts, etc).

Tangential Question: What other perennial Board favorite is associated with abdominal pain, GI bleeding, and eosinophilia? There is a vignette on this elsewhere in the book—stay tuned.

Here's the Point!

Vasculopath + Anemia + "Needle-Shaped Clefts" on Mucosal Biopsy = Cholesterol Embolization to the GI Tract

Vignette 6: Young Man with Severe Vomiting

A 48-year-old man presents to the emergency department with a 12-hour history of recurrent, severe retching and vomiting after binge drinking. He complains of a sharp "stabbing" pain over his precordium radiating to his left midaxillary line diffusely. He has no hematemesis, melena, or hematochezia. Nasogastric lavage causes significant discomfort and is aborted.

His vital signs are as follows: RR=24; Oxygen Saturation=93% on room air; BP=132/86 (not orthostatic); Pulse=110 and regular. On exam he appears tachypneic and in mild distress. His right lung is clear to auscultation throughout, and his left lung reveals diminished breath sounds at the base with dullness to percussion overlying the affected area. There is no subcutaneous crepitus over the precordium or neck.

After 30 minutes of observation he becomes progressively more short of breath and now has radiation of his pain into his left neck. A chest x-ray reveals fluid in the left lung. Shortly after the film is shot he vomits blood.

▶ **What is going on?**

▶ **What is the next step in management?**

Vignette 6: Answer

This is Boerhaave's Syndrome, or a transmural laceration of the distal esophagus. This may be relatively straightforward to you, which is good. But the temptation is to confuse this for a simple case of Mallory Weiss tear and to perform upper endoscopy. Boerhaave's is actually a form of Mallory Weiss tear in which the tear is transmural. Anything short of a transmural tear is simply a Mallory Weiss tear without perforation.

When present, transmural lacerations are classically associated with a left-sided effusion, a result of the asymmetric orientation of the distal esophagus as it bends into the stomach (although right-sided effusions could certainly occur). Once it becomes advanced, there may be mediastinal air on a standard chest film, and evidence of subcutaneous crepitus on physical examination. Urgent surgery is generally required in the setting of Boerhaave's given its high mortality rate.

I always remember 1 case of Boerhaave's, in particular, I saw as a first year fellow. I was called to evaluate a patient with purported upper GI bleeding thought to be from a Mallory Weiss tear. The ER casually admitted the patient to the floor, convinced that his young age (he was 28) and good health warranted an unmonitored bed. The team called me to report the case, and offered reassurance that the patient was doing fine and was "just another drinker who threw up too much." I figured I had time to catch lunch, and ran to the cafeteria to grab a bite.

By the time I got to the patient's bed, he seemed a bit short of breath. He was using his intercostal muscles to breathe, which seemed odd for such a young and healthy guy. I did my usual exam of his neck, and immediately felt the "snap" and "crackle" of subcutaneous air beneath my fingertips. He had crepitus. My heart sank. This guy was in trouble. There shouldn't be air in his skin. I shouldn't have eaten lunch. Time to call thoracic surgery.

Why might this be tested? Because it is an uncommon presentation (perforation) of a common condition (Mallory Weiss tear), and they will want to ensure you can tell the difference between a mere GI bleeding urgency and a surgical emergency.

Here's the Point!

Hematemesis + Subcutaneous Air + Left-Sided Effusion = Mallory Weiss Tear with Boerhaave's Syndrome. Call surgery immediately!

Vignette 7: AIDS Diarrhea

A 48-year-old man with AIDS, CD4=136, presents with a 3-month history of large volume watery stools and low-grade fevers. He complains of right lower quadrant abdominal pain. Outside labs revealed an MCV of 103 and stool studies that were negative for *C. difficile*, and ova and parasites.

You perform enteroscopy and colonoscopy that are macroscopically unremarkable. Biopsies of the proximal jejunum are pictured (Figure 7-1).

Figure 7-1. Biopsies of the proximal jejunum. (Courtesy of Wilfred Weinstein, MD, David Geffen School of Medicine at UCLA.)

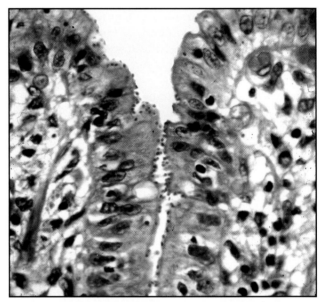

▶ *What is the diagnosis?*

▶ *Why the elevated MCV?*

▶ *Why the lower abdominal pain?*

Vignette 7: Answer

This is cryptosporidiosis with terminal ileal involvement. *Cryptosporidium* accounts for up to 10% of HIV-related diarrhea, so it is always a good bet to keep this organism in mind whenever a patient with AIDS presents with watery stool. It is most common when the CD4 count falls below 180. It is spread thorough drinking water. It can affect immunocompetent patients as well, as described in several published outbreaks of this agent (most famous is an outbreak in a college in Milwaukee, first described in the *New England Journal of Medicine* in 1993—okay, admittedly not on Boards!).

Notably, *Cryptosporidium* can involve both the biliary tract (and lead to cholecystitis) and the terminal ileum. The latter can lead to vitamin B12 deficiency and macrocytic anemia. Low-grade fevers are common. Endoscopic biopsy classically reveals trophozoites that are on the surface layer—not intracellular.

There are no consistently effective treatments, and the usual approach is to treat the underlying HIV itself and to use antidiarrheal agents as needed (often requires tincture of opium). However, data indicate that nitazoxanide demonstrates promise as an effective agent, particularly when the CD4 count is still above 50. In immunocompetent patients the infection is typically cleared without active treatment.

Why might this be tested? Because the Board examiners seem to love anything that affects the terminal ileum. Plus, it is a safe bet that there will be questions about AIDS-related opportunistic infections. This vignette merges both high-yield areas.

Clinical Threshold Alert: Cryptosporidiosis most likely when CD4<180.

Here's the Point!

Fever + Diarrhea + B12 Deficiency = Sure, could be Crohn's. But could also be Cryptosporidiosis

Vignette 8: Recurrent Abdominal Pain and Lip Swelling

An 18-year-old man presents to the emergency department with severe diffuse abdominal pain. The pain came on suddenly while he was sleeping. He has a history of recurrent, irregular episodes of similar diffuse abdominal pain. He reports a family history of a similar condition. Examination of his face reveals swelling of his lip, and CT scan of the abdomen reveals diffuse small bowel wall thickening.

▶ *What is the most likely diagnosis?*

▶ *What else might be in the differential diagnosis?*

▶ *What is the treatment?*

Vignette 8: Answer

This is hereditary angioedema. Hereditary angioedema is an autosomal dominant disease marked by a deficiency in C1 esterase activity. The absence or reduction in C1 esterase leads to unabated complement activation and subsequent inflammation.

Clinically, hereditary angioedema may present with episodic bouts of acute, diffuse, and severe abdominal pain. They may be associated with peripheral and visceral edema and swelling. If you have ever seen a case, you can't easily forget it: severe pain, writhing in bed in extremis, similar to a bowel infarction. Attacks are classically triggered by initiation of an ACE inhibitor, although they may be associated with other stressors (eg, viral illness), or may simply be spontaneous and unpredictable.

The differential diagnosis is quite limited, particularly when there is a family history and characteristics findings (episodic abdominal pain with peripheral and visceral edema). Familial Mediterranean Fever (FMF) is often in the differential because it also runs in families and presents with episodic severe abdominal pain (see Vignette 93). But FMF is not associated with peripheral and visceral edema. Crohn's Disease can run in families, present with episodic abdominal pain, and be associated with lip involvement (granulomatous, not edematous). In the most extreme form, Crohn's can present with the so-called Melkersson-Rosenthal Syndrome, in which patients have recurrent tongue swelling, a fissured tongue, facial paralysis, and noncaseating granulomas of the tongue in association with facial Crohn's. But its similarities to hereditary angioedema end there, and the 2 conditions should be easily distinguished.

Acute abdominal attacks of hereditary angioedema can be treated with infusions of C1 esterase concentrates. Long-term prophylaxis is with danazol.

Why might this be tested? Because it is rare and treatable. Also because there is a nice clinicopathologic correlation. Finally, it can be linked to intriguing pictures, like a swollen lip or diffusely swollen small bowel on CT.

Here's the Point!

Recurrent Abdominal Pain + Family History + Visceral & Peripheral Edema = Hereditary Angioedema (probably not FMF)

Vignettes 9-16: GI/Dermatology Overlaps

Gastroenterologists spend a lot of time interpreting lumps, bumps, polyps, ulcers, and other mucosal-based abnormalities of the luminal digestive tract. In essence, gastroenterology is the study of "endodermatology." But many conditions have both endo- and "exo-dermatologic" features, so you should be able to recognize the outward signs of internal digestive disorders. Below is a collection of classic GI/Dermatology overlaps. Read each vignette, and then answer the embedded questions at the end of each vignette.

9. A 72-year-old man presents with a dark, velvety rash on his anterior neck, right axilla, and bilateral hands. He has lost 15 pounds unintentionally over the last month. His primary care physician refers him to you because labs reveal a microcytic, iron-deficiency anemia. He had a normal screening colonoscopy 3 years prior to this evaluation. There is no family history of GI malignancy. He is not diabetic, and his body mass index is 28. What is the name of the skin lesion? What is the most likely GI diagnosis? Why is it relevant that he is not diabetic or obese?

10. A 56-year-old male alcoholic is admitted for acute pancreatitis. The inpatient course is prolonged, and the patient ultimately requires total parenteral nutrition (TPN) for nutritional support. After 1 week of TPN he develops diarrhea and erythematous, scaling, vesicopustular plaques on his legs and face. What is the diagnosis and treatment?

11. An 80-year-old woman presents to her primary care physician with an outbreak of pruritic seborrheic keratoses. She has not previously had seborrheic keratoses despite her advanced age. Her physician refers the patient to you for pan-endoscopy. Why?

12. A 23-year-old man presents with acute upper GI tract hemorrhage and severe diffuse abdominal pain that culminates in a bowel perforation. He has a history of fragile skin with easy bruisability, hyperextensible joints, and vascular aneurysms. What is the underlying diagnosis?

13. A 32-year-old woman presents with acute pancreatitis. She has no history of alcohol intake or gallstones, and ultrasound does not reveal evidence of new gallstone disease. She previously had abdominal pain and was diagnosed with "peritonitis" of unclear etiology. On review of systems, she describes recent hair loss and skin rashes. Exam reveals evidence of alopecia and multiple erythematous plaques with overlying adherent scales extending into hair follicles. These lesions are most prevalent on her face, neck, and scalp. What is the most likely diagnosis?

14. A 60-year-old woman presents with new-onset diabetes mellitus, anorexia, weight loss, and diarrhea. She developed a rash 2 years prior to the onset of these symptoms. The rash has returned intermittently since it first appeared. The rash usually begins under the folds of her breast or buttocks, and then spreads, becomes raised, blisters, and crusts over. This sequence occurs over a 1 to 2 week period. On exam there is evidence of erythematous lesions in her groin, thighs, and buttocks, along with glossitis, dystrophic nails, and angular stomatitis. What is the name of the erythematous skin lesion? What is the underlying diagnosis?

15. A 38-year-old man presents with 1 day of nausea, vomiting, and hematemesis. He is evaluated in the emergency department where a nasogastric lavage reveals coffee grounds in the aspirate but no active bleeding. His vital signs are stable. On further examination, you identify "pebbly papules" on his neck, antecubital fossae, and axillae. The pebbles appear to coalesce into plaques in several areas. There are xanthelasma on his eyelids. In a secondary check of his medical records, you find that a recent history and physical from ophthalmology reported "angioid streaks" on his retina bilaterally. Endoscopy is planned but has not yet been performed. What is this condition? Is this inherited?

16. A 30-year-old man develops recurrent right-lower-quadrant abdominal pain. Subsequent colonoscopy reveals diffuse apthous ulcerations in the terminal ileum. He is presumptively diagnosed with Crohn's Disease and treated with mesalamine, which does not improve his symptoms. He is treated with budesonide as a second-line agent, again without improvements. While being treated, he develops oral and scrotal ulcerations, along with anterior uveitis. He is started on steroids, which improves his abdominal pain and mucocutaneous lesions. What is the underlying diagnosis?

Vignettes 9-16: Answers

9. This is acanthosis nigricans, probably from an underlying gastric malignancy. Acanthosis nigricans is a velvety rash typically found in the nape of the neck, axillae, and hands. It is most commonly seen in patients with the metabolic syndrome, characterized by glucose intolerance and obesity, among other hallmarks. But the skin lesion is also a paraneoplastic phenomenon, and gastric malignancy is the most common underlying malignancy in the setting of acanthosis nigricans. Other common malignancies include hepatocellular cancer and lung cancer.

The fact that this patient is neither diabetic nor obese suggests the lesion is less likely from metabolic syndrome, and more likely from an underlying malignancy. The finding of iron deficiency anemia strongly suggests a gastric malignancy. Hepatocellular cancer is less likely to lead to iron deficiency anemia, although it too could potentially lead to bleeding through the rare mechanism of hemobilia (more of a "fun fact" than a relevant factor in this case).

Here's the Point!

Black Velvety Rash + Lack of Metabolic Syndrome = Possible Malignancy. Think gastric and hepatocellular in particular.

10. This is zinc deficiency. Zinc deficiency is especially common among alcoholics (beer drinkers, in particular, as beer has virtually no zinc), and can also develop in patients on total parenteral nutrition (TPN) therapy if zinc is not added to the formulation. It has also been described in patients with Crohn's Disease. Zinc may also be sequestered in the liver during episodes of physiological stress, including trauma, infection, or other acute systemic inflammatory conditions. In these instances there is not a true deficiency, but a functional deficiency as the zinc is maldistributed.

Zinc deficiency leads to a characteristic acral-predominant skin lesion that appears as an erythematous, scaling, vesicopustular plaque on the legs and face. It is also associated with diarrhea, as occurred here. The lesions can rapidly improve with appropriate zinc supplementation.

Here's the Point!

Diarrhea + Erythematous Scaling Plaques on Legs and Face + TPN, Alcoholism, or Crohn's = Zinc Deficiency

11. This is the sign of Leser-Trelat which is a sudden, extensive outbreak of seborrheic keratoses. Seborrheic keratoses are benign and common. However, when they appear as a dramatic, extensive, and simultaneous outbreak, then it may be a paraneoplastic syndrome from underlying visceral or pulmonary malignancy. The most common cancers associated with the sign include colon, gastric, liver, pancreas, and lung. Pan-endoscopy is warranted, particularly if there is concurrent acanthosis nigricans.

Here's the Point!

Sudden Outbreak of Seborrheic Keratoses = Think Underlying GI Malignancy

12. This is Ehlers-Danlos Syndrome. Ehlers-Danlos syndrome includes several subtypes, all of which have in common a defect in type III collagen. This leads to skin fragility, hypermobility of joints, and hyperelasticity of tissue. The most serious cardiovascular complication is aortic root dilatation and rupture. Ehlers-Danlos syndrome Type IV, in particular, is associated with splanchnic arterial aneurysms, GI bleeding, and bowel perforations.

Here's the Point!

Joint Hypermobility and Bowel Trouble = Think Ehlers-Danlos Syndrome

13. This is systemic lupus erythematosis (SLE). SLE is one of those conditions that affect virtually every organ system, and the GI tract is no exception. GI manifestations of lupus include peritonitis, pancreatitis (as seen here), and colitis. This patient has evidence of discoid lupus, which presents with erythematous plaques and follicular plugging. A simple malar rash would have been too easy!

Here's the Point!

Woman with Abdominal Pain + Rash or Hair Loss = Think Lupus

14. This is glucagonoma with necrolytic migratory erythema. Glucagonomas are neuroendocrine tumors that give rise to a unique syndrome of dermatitis, glucose intolerance (or frank diabetes), and weight loss. They are most commonly found in the pancreatic head and often metastasize. The characteristic skin rash often predates the diagnosis of glucagonoma by many years. It presents initially as erythematous patches in the intertriginous regions like the buttocks, thighs, and groin. It then runs through a characteristic 1 to 2 week cycle of lateral expansion, bullae formation, rupturing, and crusting. The lesions can leave hyperpigmented patches upon healing. The cycle may repeat itself several times. Other manifestations of glucagonoma include dystrophic nails, angular stomatitis, and glossitis. Weight loss is prominent, probably because of the catabolic effects of glucagon, coupled with inadequate nutrient assimilation from the inhibition of insulin.

Diabetes
Dematiti
Weight loss

Here's the Point!

> **Dermatitis (Necrolytic Migratory Erythema) + Glucose Intolerance + Weight Loss = Glucagonoma**

15. This is pseudoxanthoma elasticum (PXE). PXE is a disorder characterized by abnormal elastic tissue deposition and calcifications. It is a sporadic, autosomal recessive condition (although autosomal dominant forms have been described). The underlying defect is a mutation in the ABCC6 gene on chromosome 16. PXE classically involves the skin, eyes, and cardiovascular and GI systems. Dermatologically, PXE is characterized by 2 to 5 mm yellowish papules, which may coalesce into plaques. This gives the so-called "plucked chicken skin" appearance of PXE.

Gastrointestinal bleeding can occur from mucosal-based lesions in the foregut related to the abnormal tissue deposition in the gastric arteries. Cardiovascularly, PXE is characterized by accelerated atherosclerosis, although that is probably not a GI-Board fact.

Fundoscopy reveals angioid streaks, which also happen to be associated with Paget's Disease (that is another "pearl": angioid streaks + ↑ALP = Paget's).

Here's the Point!

> **GI Bleeding + "Plucked Chicken Skin" = Pseudoxanthoma Elasticum**

16. This is Bechet's Disease. Bechet's is a vasculitis associated with a range of mucocutaneous lesions, including oral ulcers, genital ulcers, and anterior uveitis, among others. The condition usually falls within the purview of rheumatology, but gastroenterologists should be familiar with its GI manifestations. Bechet's can mimic Crohn's disease because it often affects the terminal ileum, and may present with apthous ulcerations in the intestinal lumen and mouth. Bechet's can lead to intestinal perforations in severe cases, so patients with Bechet's are occasionally misdiagnosed as having Crohn's Disease, as happened here. As an aside, other vasculidites that can affect the GI tract include Churg-Strauss Syndrome, Henoch-Schonlein Purpura, Polyarteritis Nodosa, and Lupus.

Here's the Point!

**Terminal Ileal Apthous Ulcers + Oral and Genital Ulcers =
Think Bechet's Syndrome**

Vignettes 17-22: Ascitic Fluid Interpretations

This is really more like 6 vignettes rolled up into 1. Each row below represents a separate cirrhotic patient with ascites. In each case there is a PMN count from the fluid, results of a culture (positive vs. negative for typical spontaneous bacterial peritonitis [SBP] organisms), and presence vs. absence of typical SBP symptoms (abdominal pain, fevers, progressive encephalopathy, etc). For each case, fill in the diagnosis (eg, "SBP") and whether or not appropriate antibiotic treatment is warranted.

Vignette	PMN Count	Ascitic Fluid Culture	SBP Symptoms	Diagnosis	Treat? (Yes or No)
17	490	+	Yes		
18	490	–	Yes		
19	50	+	Yes		
20	50	+	No		
21	99	–	No		
22	400	+	No		

Vignettes 17-22: Answers

The answers are provided in the table below.

Vignette	PMN Count	Ascitic Fluid Culture	SBP Symptoms	Diagnosis	Treat? (Yes or No)
17	490	+	Yes	SBP	Yes
18	490	–	Yes	CNNA	Yes
19	50	+	Yes	NNBA	Yes
20	50	+	No	NNBA	+/–
21	99	–	No	Normal	No
22	400	+	No	SBP	Yes

(SBP=Spontaneous Bacterial Peritonitis;CNNA=Culture Negative Neutrocytic Ascites; NNBA=Non-Neutrocytic Bacterascites).

Ascitic fluid in cirrhosis can be classified according to the algorithm in Figure 17-1. The first decision point is whether the PMN count is above or below 250. If above, treatment with appropriate antibiotics (typically a third-generation cephalosporin like cefotaxime) should be initiated, regardless of the culture results or symptoms.

The second decision point is whether the culture yields typical SBP organisms, such as *E. coli*, Klebsiella, and Pneumococcus. When the PMN count exceeds 250 and the culture is positive, then the diagnosis is obviously SBP. When the count exceeds 250 but the culture is negative, then the diagnosis is culture negative neutrocytic ascites, or CNNA. This may be a false negative culture, or a partly treated SBP. In any event, CNNA should be treated just like SBP, regardless of presence vs absence of symptoms. If the PMN count is below 250 and there is a positive culture, this is termed non-neutrocytic bacterascites (NNBA).

There has been controversy about how best to treat this (controversy alert!— probably not on exam!), and some defer to presence vs absence of symptoms in deciding whether to treat.

Finally, if there is a PMN count <250 and the culture is negative, then there is no treatment rendered.

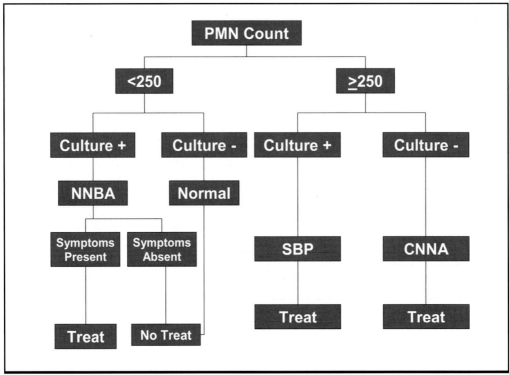

Figure 17-1. Algorithmic approach to ascitic fluid interpretation in cirrhosis.

Why might this be tested? Because this is a common clinical problem that lends itself to a neat diagnostic and therapeutic algorithm (with the exception of NNBA management).

Clinical Threshold Alert: Treat for SBP if the ascitic fluid PMN count exceeds 250.

Here's the Point!

Treat CNNA like SBP. Remember 250 PMN Thresholds for SBP.

Vignette 23: Dysphagia and Thick Skin

A 58-year-old man is referred from his primary care physician for progressive dysphagia. The dysphagia began 3 months ago, and at first was associated only with solid foods. He subsequently developed increasingly severe symptoms, and 1 month ago developed intolerance of liquids as well as solids. He lost 18 pounds unintentionally over the 3 months since developing dysphagia. He also noted dramatic thickening of the skin on both his hands and the soles of both feet at about the time his dysphagia began.

On examination he is thin, has temporal wasting, and appears cachectic. Oral exam reveals leukoplakia on the buccal mucosa. He is noted to have keratoderma on both hands and the soles of both feet. Rectal exam reveals guaiac positive stool.

▸ *What is this condition?*

▸ *Is this inherited?*

▸ *What is the GI association?*

▸ *What is endoscopy likely to reveal?*

Vignette 23: Answer

This is Tylosis, otherwise known as Howel-Evans Syndrome. Tylosis is an autosomal dominant disorder characterized by hyperkeratinization of the palms and soles. It is extremely rare (thus on Boards). This condition has a high association with cancer, and 95% of patients develop cancer by age 70. Gastrointestinal associations include oral leukoplakia and, more importantly, squamous cell carcinoma of the esophagus.

Endoscopy is warranted to evaluate for cancer in this particular patient. It is recommended to begin surveillance for esophageal cancer starting at age 30, with follow-up endoscopy every 1 to 3 years thereafter. However, this recommendation is not very evidence-based, and is not really set in stone—thus, unlikely to be tested. But you should certainly know this entity, in any event.

Why might this be tested? Because it is practically the rarest thing ever! And because the Boards love questions on dermatological manifestations of GI disorders (in this case, a GI manifestation of a dermatological disorder, really). Finally, expect to see 1 or 2 questions on squamous cell cancer—the neoplastic "stepchild" of the esophagus. There is always such an emphasis on adenocarcinoma of the esophagus, but it is important to know the basics about squamous cell as well.

Here's the Point!

Keratoderma of Palms and Soles + Dysphagia =
Tylosis with Esophageal Squamous Cell Carcinoma

Vignette 24: All Plugged Up

You are evaluating a 61-year-old woman who presents with a chief complaint of constipation. She has 3 BMs weekly, and all of her BMs are associated with prolonged defecation and severe straining. On occasion she even needs to manually disimpact her stool in order to "loosen it up." She describes her stools as "hard" and "lumpy," "like little rocks." Her symptoms have not improved with stool softeners, fiber, or laxatives.

She recently underwent colonoscopy to evaluate for structural lesions, and it revealed internal hemorrhoids but no other significant findings. Her CBC, electrolytes, glucose, and TSH are all normal. She is not receiving any medications that could promote constipation. You decide to perform anorectal manometry with balloon expulsion. As the patient bears down to attempt expulsion, the manometric tracing in Figure 24-1 is produced.

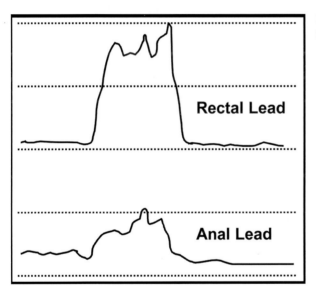

Figure 24-1. Anorectal manometry tracing during balloon expulsion.

Rectal Lead

Anal Lead

▶ *What is the diagnosis?*

▶ *What is the treatment?*

Vignette 24: Answer

This is pelvic dyssynergia, or functional anorectal outlet obstruction. During a normal BM, pressure in the rectum increases while pressure in the anal canal decreases. The anal sphincters are striated muscles under voluntary control. In order to easily evacuate a stool, the anal sphincter should relax to reduce the physical barrier to expulsion. But some people are literally "anal retentive." They keep their external anal sphincter paradoxically "tight" at the very moment when they should be relaxing.

The tip-off on anorectal manometry is a paradoxical increase in the anal pressure that correlates with the increase in rectal pressure. The increase in rectal pressure is a normal consequence of the Valsalva maneuver, and is the initiating event for defecation. This is accompanied by a relaxation of the puborectalis sling, which allows a straightening of the anorectal angle. The final part of a normal reflex is the relaxation of the anal sphincter, which is normally detected with a decrease—not increase—in the anal pressure. In this case the pressure in the anal canal is going up, not down. That is like trying to squeeze toothpaste out of the tube while keeping the cap on. You have got to take the cap off to get the toothpaste out. Stool is no different.

This is probably more common than we think. Pelvic dyssynergia can be detected by a standard balloon expulsion test, in which a patient has a rectal balloon instilled with 50 to 60 cc of water, and then has 2 minutes to expel the balloon while on a commode (easier said than done, even for nondyssynergic patients). If the balloon cannot be expelled within 2 minutes, it suggests potential dyssynergic defecation. Anorectal manometry is the gold standard for diagnosis, as described above. Another approach to diagnosis is to use a radioopaque marker study (Sitzmark study). If the markers collect in the rectum without being expelled, then it provides further evidence for possible anorectal outlet obstruction.

The definitive treatment for pelvic dyssynergia is biofeedback therapy, in which patients learn to literally relax their external anal sphincter during defecation—a process that typically requires several sessions with active coaching and real-time feedback regarding sphincter tone. Traditional laxative therapy is not very effective in this condition, since the problem is not one of motility, but of outlet obstruction.

Why might this be tested? This is classic manometric pattern: 1 of the Big Four. You should know all of the Big Four: Diffuse Esophageal Spasm, Nutcracker Esophagus, Achalasia (and vigorous achalasia), and Pelvic Dyssynergia. Examples of the other Big Four come later (see Vignettes 102-109).

Here's the Point 1

Pelvic dyssynergia = Trying to poop while holding it in at the same time. You've got to take the cap off the tube to squeeze out the toothpaste!

Here's the Point 2

For manometry and the Boards, don't go nuts memorizing complex patterns and mastering nuance. Start by knowing The Big Four:

1. Diffuse Esophageal Spasm (DES)
2. Nutcracker Esophagus
3. Achalasia (and vigorous achalasia)
4. Pelvic Dyssynergia

Vignette 25: Integument Gone Wild (and polyps too!)

A 62-year-old woman is referred to you after multiple polyps were found on screening flexible sigmoidoscopy. The polyps were not biopsied. She is sent to you for colonoscopic evaluation.

On review of systems, you learn that she has been progressively losing her hair over the last 6 months, and that she has developed patches of hyperpigmented skin on her face and soles of her feet. She also complains of recurrent loose stools, but no abdominal pain.

On examination she is found to have alopecia and dystrophic fingernails. Review of her labs reveals an albumin of 2.8. Her other lab values are unremarkable. She undergoes colonoscopy, which reveals scattered polyps throughout the colon along with a bizarre appearance of subepithelial speckled hemorrhages and lymphedema throughout the visualized colon, as pictured. Biopsies are pending.

Figure 25-1. Patient's colon. (Courtesy of Binh Pham, MD, David Geffen School of Medicine at UCLA.)

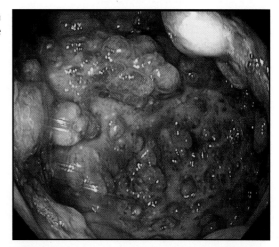

Figure 25-2. Patient's fingernails. (Courtesy of Binh Pham, MD, David Geffen School of Medicine at UCLA.)

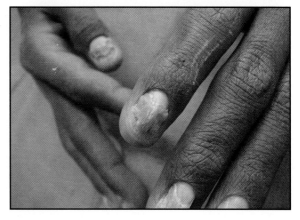

▶ *What is the most likely diagnosis?*

▶ *Is this inherited?*

Vignette 25: Answer

Autosomal Recessive !

This is Cronkhite-Canada Syndrome. Cronkhite-Canada is a noninherited condition characterized by gastric, enteric, and colonic hamartomatous polyps. Other GI manifestations include protein-losing enteropathy and associated malabsorptive diarrhea, although the mechanism for this remains unclear (I'll leave the treatise on this complex and uncertain condition to other books). Curiously, the condition is associated with integument abnormalities, including alopecia and dystrophic fingernails. It is important to keep in mind that Cronkhite-Canada is different from other hamartomatous syndromes such as Peutz-Jegher's Syndrome, Tuberous Sclerosis, Juvenile Polyposis, and Cowden's Syndrome, since it is not inherited. Each of the other syndromes is autosomal dominant. We don't know much about Cronkhite-Canada Syndrome, and there is currently no consistently effective treatment, so questions about directed treatment are unlikely to appear.

As an aside, if in doubt, it is usually a good bet to assume an inherited condition on the GI Boards is autosomal dominant. Just think about it. Nearly every "Board-type" inherited condition in GI is autosomal dominant. Here is a list, in no particular order, of autosomal dominant disorders with GI manifestations: Cowden's Syndrome, Hereditary Angioedema, Tylosis, Multiple Endocrine Neoplasia Type I (MEN I), FAP, Peutz-Jegher's Syndrome, Neurofibromatosis, Juvenile Polyposis, Osler Weber Rendu disease, Blue Rubber Bleb Nevus Syndrome (BRBNS), Inherited Intestinal Lymphangiectasia, Gardner's Syndrome, HNPCC syndrome, Von Hippel Lindau, and Tuberous Sclerosis. Obviously there are a bunch of autosomal recessive conditions you need to know about (eg, Hereditary Hemochromatosis, Wilson's Disease, Abetalipoproteinemia), but if in doubt, there seems to be more autosomal dominant than recessive conditions in the Board eligible world of GI and Hepatology.

Why might this be tested? Because it is a curiosity. Seriously, nobody knows how this condition comes about, but it does happen. The images on the previous page are photos taken at Harbor-UCLA by our fellows and faculty—everyone sat around stymied by what they were seeing. So you just need to know about this. And, once again, the Boards love questions that test knowledge about dermatological manifestations of GI diseases, and this is yet another in a long series.

Here's the Point!

Losing Hair + Nail Trouble + Polyps = Cronkhite-Canada Syndrome

Vignette 26: Dyspepsia with Thickened Gastric Folds

A 22-year-old woman is referred for dyspepsia. Her symptoms began 8 months ago, and were marked by epigastric discomfort and progressive early satiety. She has recurrent nausea and vomiting, progressive weight loss, and recently developed lower extremity edema. She has not experienced subjective fevers, chills, or sweats.

Her primary care physician treated her with double-dose proton pump inhibitor (PPI) therapy, but there was no improvement in her symptoms after 8 weeks of treatment. Pertinent positives on examination include moderate epigastric tenderness to palpation and lower extremity pitting edema. Pertinent negatives include lack of fever, no abdominal masses, and no lymphadenopathy.

Her primary care physician previously ordered an upper GI series that revealed diffusely thickened gastric folds but no discrete mass. Her gastrin was elevated at 230. With a secretin challenge, the gastrin rose to 300. Her albumin is 2.7.

You perform upper endoscopy. Key findings are pictured in Figure 26-1. Biopsies are pending.

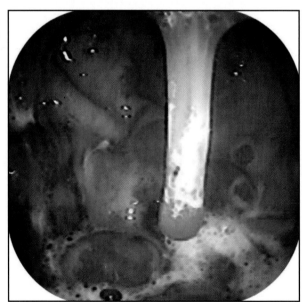

Figure 26-1. (Courtesy of Wilfred Weinstein, MD, David Geffen School of Medicine, UCLA.)

▶ *What is this condition?*

▶ *What specific abnormality may be seen on biopsy of the gastric body?*

▶ *How can this be treated?*

Vignette 26: Answer

This is Menetrier's Disease. This is a fascinating condition marked by tortuous gastric mucosal folds that characteristically spare the antrum. The folds can be very dramatic, as pictured, and coupled with "stalactites" of mucous hanging from the ceiling. The histology classically reveals "corkscrew" foveolar hyperplasia (thus lots of mucous production) and a relative lack of oxyntic gland mucosa (Figure 26-2).

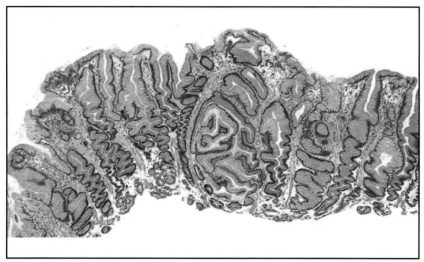

Figure 26-2. Characteristic "corkscrew" of foveolar hyperplasia of Menetrier's Disease. (Courtesy of Wilfred Weinstein, MD, David Geffen School of Medicine at UCLA.)

Antrum NOT involved

The etiology of Menetrier's remains largely unknown, although it has been linked to CMV and *H. pylori*. But the jury is out on the strength of this relationship, and the linkage is stronger in children than adults. It is also associated with lymphocytic gastritis (see Vignette 34), hypoalbuminemic protein-losing enteropathy, and associated edema.

It is important to become familiar with the differential diagnosis of thickened gastric folds, since many other conditions can masquerade as Menetrier's, and vice versa. Gastric lymphoma, in particular, can present with recurrent nausea, vomiting, and thickened gastric folds. The lack of "B symptoms" in this vignette argues against lymphoma. Zollinger Ellison Syndrome (ZES) can also present with dyspepsia, diarrhea, and thickened gastric folds. The mildly elevated gastrin suggests ZES, but is not in the usual range for this syndrome (1000+). The gastrin elevation is likely from the concurrent use of double-dose proton-pump inhibitor (PPI) therapy.

However, to help distinguish a PPI effect from possible underlying ZES, a secretin stimulation test can be administered. With ZES the gastrin should rise by at least 200 units after injection of a standard dose of secretin. Here the gastrin rose by only 70 points (from 200 to 270), indicating a low likelihood of underlying ZES (see Vignettes 29-33 for more on gastrin physiology).

Treatment of Menetrier's typically includes eradication of *H. pylori* if present. Although eradication is highly effective for mucosa-associated lymphoid tissue (MALT) and lymphocytic gastritis, it is less effective for reversing Menetrier's.

More recently (and this is now established enough to be a Board question, in my judgment), anti-epidermal growth factor receptor antibodies (ie, cetuximab) have been shown to be highly effective in many cases of Menetrier's. Menetrier's is premalignant and is sometimes a forerunner of gastric lymphoma and gastric adenocarcinoma. Surveillance should be performed, although a precise schedule has not been widely established.

Why might this be tested? Because Menetrier's is premalignant and should not be dismissed as a mere curiosity. Also, this condition provides a great opportunity to test on a range of other conditions that can lead to thickened gastric folds, such as lymphoma and ZES. So it requires that you know about a range of topics, including gastrin and secretin stimulation test interpretation, dyspepsia management (ie, when to perform endoscopy), and histopathology, among others.

Clinical Threshold Alert: Secretin stimulation test is positive if there is greater than 200 unit increase in gastrin levels.

Rx: HP eradication, anti-EGF therapy

Here's the Point!

Thick Gastric Folds + Diarrhea + Low Albumin + Edema = Menetrier's

Vignette 27: Stroke and Liver Disease

You are consulted to evaluate a 40-year-old woman who was admitted to the hospital for an acute stroke, and who was found to have abnormal liver tests on admission laboratories. Upon admission, neuroimaging revealed that the stroke resulted from a cervical artery dissection.

The patient is now aphasic, and no past medical history is available. Her vital signs are unremarkable. She has not been hypotensive at any time during the hospital course. Her physical exam reveals mildly icteric sclerae, spider angiomata on the anterior chest, and mild pitting edema. She has no evidence of heart failure.

Abnormal lab tests include: albumin=2.9; INR=1.3; total bilirubin=2.8; AST=80; and ALT=109. Her ferritin and iron saturation are normal. Toxicology screen, alcohol level, and acetaminophen level were normal at the time of admission.

You decide to perform a liver biopsy, which subsequently reveals periodic acid-Schiff-positive "globules" in the endoplasmic reticulum of the hepatocytes, along with bridging fibrosis.

▸ *What is this condition?*

▸ *Does the mechanism of stroke help to establish the diagnosis?*

▸ *What is the definitive treatment?*

Vignette 27: Answer

This is alpha-1 antitrypsin (A1AT) deficiency. A1AT deficiency is an autosomal codominant disorder that leads to a range of problems, including liver disease, pulmonary emphysema, panniculitis, and arterial aneurysms. The A1AT gene is on chromosome 14. A1AT is a serine protease inhibitor that normally responds as part of the acute phase reaction to combat injury and inflammation by inhibiting catabolic products of neutrophils, such as elastase.

In addition, A1AT inhibits a host of other destructive proteins, including trypsin and collagenase, and thus plays an important role in maintaining the integrity of tissues of many organs. The normal protease inhibitor (Pi) allele is called Pi*MM. The so-called Pi*ZZ allele, however, leads to extremely low levels of A1AT, whereas the Pi*MZ allele is associated with an intermediate level of deficiency. A1AT occurs in 1 in 2000 people, and thus is probably more common than we think. It is certainly not the most common inherited metabolic liver disease (that honor goes to Hereditary Hemochromatosis), but it is the most common metabolic liver disease among liver transplant recipients—the only cure for hepatic A1AT deficiency.

The liver manifestations of A1AT deficiency arise from a defect in protein secretion from the endoplasmic reticulum (ER). The A1AT proteins get "stuck" and accumulate in the hepatocyte ER, and are classically detected as periodic acid-Schiff (PAS)-positive "globules" that are "diastase-resistant." These accumulations of protein may have direct hepatotoxic effects, although the exact pathogenesis remains unclear and thus is unlikely to be the subject of a Board question. Interestingly, the disequilibrium between proteolytic enzymes and protease inhibitors has been implicated in the pathogenesis of arterial aneurysms and dissections of medium-to-large vessels. Cervical artery dissection is one of the most common arterial consequences of A1AT deficiency, although other vessels, including the aorta, can be affected.

Still, arterial dissections are relatively uncommon in A1AT. A1AT is also associated with an ulcerative, neutrophilic panniculitis. This is often found on the trunk, and can demonstrate pathergy—ie, worsening with trauma. As an aside, there is another skin lesion associated with a GI condition that classically demonstrates pathergy. It happens with IBD. You can sit on that one for now... I'll give you the answer in a few sentences.

In any event, as noted above, treatment for the liver manifestations of A1AT deficiency is transplantation. Whereas the lung form of A1AT deficiency can be treated with replacement therapy of recombinant plasma A1AT, this therapy is not indicated for liver disease. And as for that other pathergic lesion: pyoderma gangrenosum.

Why might this be tested? Because this is an unusual presentation of an unusual disorder, so it is perfect for the Boards. It is almost a guarantee that metabolic liver diseases will show up on the exam somewhere, so it should come as no surprise that A1AT deficiency may show up. But just knowing that something is on the exam does not mean you can get the question right, or even identify the diagnosis when it is sitting there right before your eyes. So dressing up Board favorites with rare presentations, like arterial dissections or panniculitis, is one technique to "cull the wheat from the chaff" amongst test takers. And examiners also love anything that stains positive for PAS! Seriously. Other PAS-positive Board favorites include Whipple's Disease and enteric MAC infections. More on those in other vignettes.

Here's the Point!

Arterial Dissection + Cirrhosis + PAS-positive Diatase Resistant globules on liver biopsy = Alpha-1 Antitrypsin Deficiency

Vignette 28: Something's in the Gallbladder

A 32-year-old woman is referred to you for evaluation of an abnormal right-upper quadrant ultrasound. She originally presented to her primary care physician with recurrent lower abdominal pain in association with abnormalities in stool frequency and form. She was diagnosed with IBS. However, she underwent a battery of diagnostic tests to rule out alternative diagnoses, all of which were normal with the exception of the ultrasound, which revealed a roughly 2-cm polypoid lesion, as pictured (Figure 28-1). There were no gallstones seen. On further questioning, you confirm that her symptoms meet Rome criteria for IBS, and that she does not have biliary type pain or other foregut symptoms.

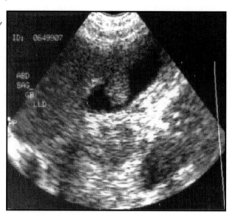

Figure 28-1. (Used with permission from Francis J. Scholz, MD, Lahey Clinic, Burlington, MA.)

▶ *What is the diagnosis?*
▶ *What is the next step to manage this?*

Vignette 28: Answer

This is a gallbladder polyp. Gallbladder polyps are a dime-a-dozen, so it is easy to blow them off as "incidentalomas" of little consequence. In fact, I have found that many GI training programs don't teach a whole lot about gallbladder polyps, and, in informal surveys, most graduating fellows have not learned the basic management principles of this very prevalent condition. Gallbladder polyps can be premalignant, so they should not be taken lightly. The issue is when, and under what circumstances, is it worth removing these polyps with a cholecystectomy. The time-tested algorithm is in Figure 28-2.

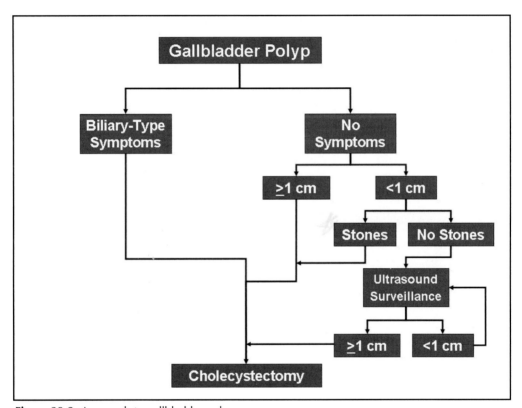

Figure 28-2. Approach to gallbladder polyps.

The first point of stratification is whether there are typical "biliary type" foregut symptoms. Lower abdominal pain, as with IBS, is not consistent with biliary-type pain. Epigastric pain, nausea, and right-shoulder or scapular pain are more suggestive. If there are biliary-type symptoms, then surgery is warranted regardless of polyp size. If there are no symptoms, then the next step is to consider polyp size.

Polyps <1 cm have a low malignancy potential and can be watched, assuming there are no concurrent stones. These are usually benign cholesterol polyps. If there are concurrent stones, then most authorities suggest proceeding to surgery regardless of polyp size. Patients with small polyps in the absence of stones undergo intermittent surveillance with follow-up ultrasound, often at 6-month intervals (although that is variable and not fully standardized). Polyps that are >1 cm carry a higher risk of malignancy and should be removed.

Although some algorithms advocate for using a 1.5 cm threshold for polyp size, most still hold the line at 1 cm. Since there is some discrepancy among sources, it would seem that the Board exam would either give you a subcentimeter polyp (a size that is not controversial), or a polyp greater than 1.5 cm. But if they threw a 1.3 cm polyp in a question, then the conservative answer would be to advocate for surgery.

In this instance the ultrasound demonstrates a polyp (note the absence of an echoic shadow, thus arguing against a stone). Because the polyp is nearly 2 cm in size, surgery is warranted, even though there are no biliary-type symptoms. Of note, EUS has gained prominence in helping to determine malignant potential, but EUS findings have not yet been formally included in most management algorithms, making a detailed question about the role of EUS in gallbladder polyps unlikely.

Why might this be tested? Examiners love polyps. You name the GI organ, and the Board may well give you a question about a polyp in that organ. And since biliary questions make up 8% of the exam, there is a reasonable chance that a question on gallbladder polyps will pop up sooner or later.

Clinical Threshold Alert: Gallbladder polyp >1 cm needs to be removed.

Here's the Point!

> **Gallbladder Polyp + Biliary Pain OR >1 cm size OR Stones = Cholecystectomy**

Vignettes 29-33: Gastrin Craziness

The table below displays 6 different acid-secretory profiles. Below the table is a list of diseases. In the blank space beside each disease, enter a letter (A through F) for the profile that best matches that disease. Note that there are more profiles than there are diseases.

Profile	Gastrin Level	Gastrin pH	Parietal Cell Mass	Secretin Stimulation Test
A	↑	↑	↑	−
B	↑	↓	↑	+
C	↑	↑	↓	−
D	↑	↓	↑	−
E	↓	↑	↓	−
F	↑	↑	↓	+

29. Zollinger-Ellison syndrome   _____ (enter letter in space)
30. Pernicious Anemia   _____
31. Corpus *H. pylori* infection   _____
32. Antrum *H. pylori* infection   _____
33. Chronic PPI use   _____

Vignettes 29-33: Answers

This set of questions provides an excuse to cover a wide range of high-yield material pertaining to acid physiology and related conditions. So it needs a bit of detail. Buckle in, this can be painful, but it is worth it.

Gastrin is secreted by "G cells" located in the (antrum.) Gastrin is secreted in the setting of the coordinated cephalic response to eating. The vagus nerve releases acetylcholine, which in turn activates the neurocrine substance GRP. GRP acts on the G cell to stimulate the release of gastrin. In addition, the vagus acts to inhibit somatostatin-secreting D Cells, also found in the antrum. Somatostatin from D cells normally acts in a paracrine manner to inhibit gastrin release from G cells. Thus, if D cells are inhibited, then local somatostatin levels fall, and G cells are free to secrete gastrin in an unopposed manner. Over time the pH of the stomach will fall, and the intraluminal H+ ions subsequently reactivate the D cells, leading to release of somatostatin and downregulation of gastrin release. This local paracrine cycle can autoregulate intraluminal pH in a highly tuned manner.

This process is in contrast to ZES, in which there is a gastrinoma autologously secreting gastrin. The gastrinomas in ZES are typically found in the "gastrinoma triangle"—an area bordered by the junction of the cystic duct and common bile duct, the junction of the head and body of the pancreas, and the junction between the second and third parts of the duodenum. In other words, the gastrinomas are not typically in the stomach at all, so they are not subject to the usual local autoregulation. A typical profile in ZES is hypergastrinemia, hypertrophic parietal cell mass (secondary to unopposed hypergastrinemia), low intraluminal gastric pH, and a positive "secretin stimulation test," in which the injection of secretin leads to a marked jump in serum gastrin levels (positive=200 unit increase). Typical serum gastrin levels in ZES are in the 1000+ range (although lower levels may certainly occur). A similar profile is seen with chronic PPI therapy, in which the parietal cell mass becomes secondarily hypertrophic from chronic suppression of acid secretion (in other words, it is "ready to blow" under the constant smothering of the PPI). This is also associated with hypergastrinemia, just as with ZES. However, unlike ZES, with chronic PPI therapy there is hypochlorhydria, a high intraluminal gastric pH, and a negative secretin stimulation test. With chronic PPI therapy the serum gastrin levels, although elevated, are typically below the 1000 level seen in ZES. A similar picture is seen with pernicious anemia, in which autoimmune destruction of the parietal cell mass leads to an atrophic gastritis.

Another important consideration is *H. pylori* infection, of which there are 2 basic types: (1) corpus predominant, and (2) antral predominant.

The corpus-predominant form of infection is marked by diffuse colonization of the parietal cell mass in the fundus and body of the stomach. Long standing infection leads to an atrophic gastritis, similar to the picture in pernicious anemia. Thus, there is hypochlorhydria, a high intraluminal pH, and reflex hypergastrinemia. The secretin stimulation test is negative. This form of *H. pylori* infection is clinically relevant, because it has implications about whether and when to eradicate *H. pylori*. In the setting of peptic ulcer disease, it is almost always recommended to test for and treat *H. pylori*. This "test and treat" approach is also recommended for nonreflux predominant dyspepsia, which is a condition marked by recurrent abdominal pain or discomfort in the upper abdomen not associated with classic reflux symptoms (see Vignettes 121-126 for more details on dyspepsia management). However, in patients who have true acid reflux disease, there is a theoretical reason to not eradicate *H. pylori*. In particular, patients with acid reflux who also have a corpus predominant infection may be relatively protected, because the *H. pylori* exerts a hypochlorhydric effect on the stomach by "knocking out" the parietal cell mass. If *H. pylori* is eradicated after years of colonization, the parietal cell mass can rebound and, in theory, hypersecrete acid. This is the last thing someone wants who already suffers from acid reflux disease. Thus, it is often recommended to not treat *H. pylori* infections in the setting of acid reflux, unless there is another clear indication for *H. pylori* treatment (eg, peptic ulcer disease, MALT lymphoma, etc). However, even this is a bit controversial, so it may not show up on the exam after all.

The antral predominant pattern of infection is marked by diffuse colonization of the antrum, with sparing of the fundus and body. The infection preferentially affects the somatostatin-secreting D cells of the antrum, leading to a lowering of somatostatin levels in the mucosa. This interferes with the local paracrine cycle of somatostatin downregulation of G cell activity, leading to an unopposed gastrin release of the antral G cells. This leads to hypergastrinemia, hypertrophy of the parietal cell mass, hyperchlorhydria, and a low intraluminal pH. This picture is similar to ZES. However, unlike with ZES, the secretin stimulation test is normal.

So, with that background, the answers to the questions are as follows:

Zollinger-Ellison syndrome: B
Pernicious Anemia: C
Corpus *H. pylori* Infection: C
Antrum *H. pylori* Infection: D
Chronic PPI Use: A

Why might this be tested? Because this material has been the source of exam questions from the beginning of time. Or at least since 1985. You just need to know this stuff.

Clinical Threshold Alert: Secretin stimulation test positive if there is greater than 200-unit increase in gastrin levels.

ZES ↔ antral HP infxn (similar)
Pernicious anemia ↔ body HP infxn (similar profile)

Vignette 34: H. pylori *Strikes Again*

A 47-year-old woman presents to your office complaining of intermittent epigastric pain occurring at least once weekly for the last 6 months. The pain lasts approximately 30 minutes and is exacerbated with food. She has no heartburn, nausea, bloating, dysphagia, or vomiting. Her weight has been stable. She has no history of peptic ulcer disease. She has no history of fever, chills, night sweats, melena or hematochezia.

Before seeing you, she was prescribed twice-daily therapy with a PPI, but her symptoms did not improve after 8 weeks of treatment. On examination her vital signs are normal. She has no abdominal tenderness to palpation, has normal bowel sounds, and no masses are palpated. Her stool is guaiac negative. The remainder of her examination is normal.

Her laboratory tests, including complete blood count, chemistry panel, and liver tests, are unremarkable. She undergoes diagnostic upper endoscopy while still on PPI therapy. The endoscopy reveals diffuse erythema and mucosal nodularity, but no discrete lesions are identified. Biopsies reveal dense intraepithelial CD8-positive T lymphocytes throughout the antrum and oxyntic mucosa, with a density exceeding 25 lymphocytes per 100 epithelial cells. There is no evidence of *H. pylori* organisms on biopsy.

▶ **What is the most likely diagnosis?**

▶ **What is the next therapeutic step?**

Vignette 34: Answer

This is lymphocytic gastritis—a rare form of gastritis characterized by dense epithelial lymphocytic infiltration throughout the stomach (>25/100 epithelial cells). Although often asymptomatic, lymphocytic gastritis can present with typical symptoms of nonreflux predominant dyspepsia. Up to 1% of all comers with dyspepsia have underlying lymphocytic gastritis.

The etiology of lymphocytic gastritis remains uncertain, although the condition does appear related to *H. pylori* infection and celiac sprue. Recent randomized controlled trials indicate that eradication of *H. pylori* can cure between 80% and 95% of cases vs 50% receiving placebo (itself interesting, since half improve without active therapy). It is important to distinguish lymphocytic gastritis from MALT lymphoma—also known as Marginal Zone B-cell lymphoma.

Whereas lymphocytic gastritis is marked by a CD8-positive T lymphocyte infiltration, MALT lymphoma is marked by diffuse populations of B-cells that expand the lamina propria, and are associated with reactive lymphoid follicles and glandular lymphoepithelial lesions. In light of the powerful relationship between *H. pylori* and lymphocytic gastritis, it is reasonable to eradicate *H. pylori* in all comers with this condition, regardless of the results of *H. pylori* testing.

In this case the biopsies were negative, but were performed while the patient was receiving high-dose PPI therapy. Since false negative tests are common while on PPI therapy, it is premature to conclude that *H. pylori* is absent. Empiric treatment is nonetheless warranted given the high cure rate of lymphocytic gastritis in the randomized trials evaluating *H. pylori* eradication, coupled with the fact that few other effective therapies are available for this condition. It is also reasonable to conduct a screening test for celiac sprue, perhaps by checking for the presence of an antitissue transglutaminase (TTG) IgA antibody.

Why might this be tested? Because the relationship between *H. pylori* and lymphocytic gastritis is nearly cause-and-effect. Although everyone knows that *H. pylori* can cause peptic ulcers, not everyone knows this relationship. So it is low-hanging fruit for a Board question.

Clinical Threshold Alert: Need >25 lymphocytes/100 epithelial cells to confirm the diagnosis of lymphocytic gastritis.

Here's the Point!

Dyspepsia + T Cell Lymphocytic Infiltrate in Stomach = Lymphocytic Gastritis
>> Eradicate *H. pylori* <<

Vignette 35: Explosive Maroon Stools

A 78-year-old woman with a history of diabetes mellitus and atrial fibrillation presents to the emergency department with lower GI bleeding. She was in her usual state of health until 4 hours prior to admission, when she developed acute, severe, unremitting abdominal pain that woke her from sleep. Two hours later she developed explosive maroon colored stools. Upon admission, her blood pressure was 98/60 and her heart rate was 114 and irregular. Nasogastric lavage yielded clear bilious fluid. Abdominal examination revealed severe diffuse tenderness out of proportion to palpation. Rectal examination confirmed maroon output with clots. You are now called to evaluate the patient for possible urgent colonoscopy.

▶ *What is the most likely diagnosis?*

▶ *What is the most appropriate test to perform at this time?*

Vignette 35: Answer

This is acute mesenteric ischemia (AMI), likely from a superior mesenteric artery embolism (SMAE). AMI is a prevalent and often fatal condition caused by an abrupt discontinuation or abatement of blood flow from either mechanical or functional occlusion of the mesenteric vessels. The most common etiologies of AMI include SMAE, nonocclusive mesenteric ischemia, SMA thrombosis, and focal segmental ischemia. Of these, SMAE accounts for roughly 50% of all cases of AMI and is the most likely explanation in this case, particularly given the history of atrial fibrillation. The severity of SMAE is stratified by its point of arrest; "major" emboli are those proximal to the origin of the ileocolic artery and "minor" embolic are those distal to the ileocolic takeoff or in the distal SMA branches (Figure 35-1). More than a simple anatomical or academic distinction, this classification scheme provides the basis for treatment decisions. The results of emergent angiography provide information on the type of embolism, location of arrest, and presence or absence of vasoconstriction. Subsequent steps are beyond the scope of this discussion, and are really in the purview of interventional radiologists in concert with surgery (eg, when to use papaverine, when to bring to surgery, etc).

The clinical presentation of AMI caused by SMAE is rarely subtle. To the contrary, patients typically develop an acute-onset abdominal pain that escalates rapidly and persists without respite. The onset of pain is often accompanied by the abrupt and forceful evacuation of bloody stool and, when severe, progressive abdominal distension (an early sign of ischemia transitioning to infarction).

Although the rich network of anastomotic loops interconnecting the mesenteric circulation provides a temporary buffer between bowel ischemia and outright necrosis, patients with preexisting vascular disease are nonetheless susceptible to rapid infarction within as little as 6 hours. Moreover, it has long been recognized that arteriolar vasoconstriction tends to accompany AMI and acts to hasten the development of bowel infarction. Since most patients with AMI already have 1 or more significant comorbidities, the physiologic deck is stacked in favor of catastrophe once the process of AMI begins.

The physical examination may reveal dramatic rebound tenderness, guarding, absent bowel sounds, and gross abdominal distention. However, AMI more commonly presents as an insidious event with abdominal pain out of proportion to palpation. Early in the course of AMI, there may be few, if any, objective physical signs.

Laboratory findings may include a leukocytosis with a "shift to the left" and metabolic acidemia in 50% of patients. Although abdominal films may demonstrate "thumbprinting" once infarction has developed, films are often normal when the patient presents. Similarly, CT rarely detects subtle SMA abnormalities and is generally incapable of visualizing the distal splanchnic circulation. Once CT detects significant abnormalities, the clinical course is usually well advanced. This "all or none" observation for abdominal imaging suggests that the results of early images cannot be used as definitive evidence to rule out AMI. To the contrary, a normal or near normal abdominal image in the setting of overwhelming abdominal pain should increase suspicion for AMI and prompt further timely evaluation.

It is not surprising that the single most important determinant of outcomes in AMI is time to diagnosis. So urgent angiography is mandatory—not urgent colonoscopy, or even urgent surgery. The "tough part" here is not making the diagnosis of AMI—that is fairly obvious. Instead, the trick is to know that interventional radiology must be called next.

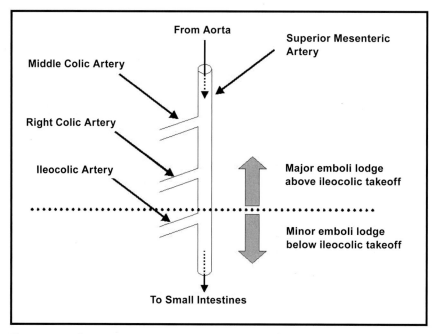

Figure 35-1. The superior mesenteric artery (SMA) and its major branches. The SMA arises from the aorta. The 3 main branches of the SMA supply the transverse colon (middle colic artery), distal ascending colon (right colic artery), and TI to proximal ascending colon (ileocolic artery). Emboli that lodge above the takeoff of the ileocolic artery are termed "major emboli," and those lodging beyond the takeoff are "minor emboli."

Why might this be tested? Because gastroenterologists miss this diagnosis way too often. We are lulled into thinking colonoscopy is warranted, but sometimes forget that SMAE might be lurking beneath, and that interventional radiology should be contacted first and foremost. Moreover, if we mess around with CT scans, imaging, surgical consults, and other forms of procrastination, then patients can die right under our eyes.

Here's the Point!

Any whiff of possible SMAE: No CT, no colonoscopy, no barium enema, no flat plate, not even surgery yet—emergent angiography for diagnosis and treatment of possible SMAE

Vignette 36: Inpatient Liver Trouble

You are consulted to evaluate a 42-year-old woman with elevated liver tests that developed as an inpatient. The patient was initially admitted to hospital 4 weeks prior to your consultation, when she underwent a bone marrow transplant for acute myelogenous leukemia. Two weeks after the transplant she developed jaundice and an elevated total bilirubin of 4. Three weeks after the transplant she developed progressive ascites and weight gain, and the bilirubin rose to 12.

Her platelet count dropped concurrently, and was most recently 38,000. Her transaminases have been mildly elevated, but never more than twice the upper limit of normal. She has not been septic during the current hospitalization, nor has she received parenteral nutrition. An abdominal ultrasound performed prior to your consultation revealed a normal gallbladder wall thickness and no evidence of gallstones or pericholecystic fluid. Doppler examination revealed a patent hepatic vein with normal flow.

On examination she has no stigmata of chronic liver disease, no rashes, and no evidence of encephalopathy, but does have shifting dullness in her abdomen and a tender, enlarged liver.

▶ **What is the most likely diagnosis?**

▶ **What are 4 other conditions that are in the differential diagnosis?**

▶ **What would a liver biopsy reveal if performed?**

Vignette 36: Answer

This is veno occlusive disease (VOD), also known as sinusoidal obstruction syndrome (SOS). VOD is marked by a nonthrombotic obstruction of the central portal venules with resulting sinusoidal dilation and congestion throughout the liver. VOD occurs from a diffuse endothelial injury of unclear etiology. Although the exact pathogenesis remains unclear, risk factors for VOD are well recognized. These include bone marrow transplantation (as in this case), chemotherapy, and azathioprine use. VOD complicates up to 50% of bone marrow transplantations, and carries up to a 70% mortality rate in that setting. Unlike graft versus host disease (GVHD), VOD tends to occur within 21 days of bone marrow transplantation.

In contrast, GVHD usually occurs later—up to 100 days after transplantation. Moreover, diffuse skin lesions often appear in GVHD, whereas skin involvement is not part of VOD. Clinically, patients with VOD typically have a conjugated hyperbilirubinemia >2 mg/dL, ascites, painful hepatomegaly, and marked weight gain over a short period. Thrombocytopenia may occur as well. Liver biopsy is not necessary to make the diagnosis, but when performed (usually through transjugular approach given the thrombocytopenia) reveals widening of the sub-endothelium in the central venules and congestion of portal sinusoids. Although there is a range of experimental therapies (not going into that here), nothing is consistently effective, making it unlikely that there will be questions about directed treatment of VOD.

In addition to GVHD, the differential diagnosis of inpatient liver test abnormalities includes sepsis, acalculous cholecystitis, drug induced liver injury, TPN, ischemic hepatitis, and Budd-Chiari, among others. In this case the vignette states that sepsis was not clinically evident. Acalculous cholecystitis is usually marked by gallbladder wall thickening and pericholecystic fluid, neither of which was documented on the abdominal ultrasound in this case.

The normal Doppler examination argues against Budd-Chiari, although it does not entirely rule it out. But given the close relationship with the bone marrow transplant, coupled with the low platelet count, VOD seems more likely than Budd-Chiari. Ischemic hepatitis seems unlikely with only moderately elevated transaminases and no history of sepsis or prolonged hypotension. She was not on TPN, ruling out TPN-related liver disease. Finally, drug-induced hepatitis must always be considered, but it does not fit this picture neatly (timing after bone marrow transplant + hepatomegaly + ascites + thrombocytopenia).

Why might this be tested? Because examiners seem to love questions about inpatient liver test abnormalities. This vignette introduces a wide differential diagnosis for inpatient liver test abnormalities, so even if VOD is not on the exam, it seems likely that one of the other masqueraders will be on it (eg, Budd-Chiari, acalculous cholecystitis, sepsis, etc).

Clinical Threshold Alert: VOD typically occurs within 21 days of a bone marrow transplant. GVHD occurs within 100 days of transplant.

Here's the Point!

Bone Marrow Transplant + Painful Hepatomegaly within 21 Days + Ascites + Weight Gain + Thrombocytopenia = Veno Occlusive Disease

Vignette 37: Abnormal Cholangiogram With Recurrent Pancreatitis

A 23-year-old woman presents with recurrent bouts of pancreatitis. She does not drink alcohol and has no history of gallstones. She reports intermittent bouts of abdominal pain and turning "yellow" for the last 10 years—generally once or twice a year. More recently she has developed a sense of "fullness" in her upper abdomen, and thinks she can feel a "knot" in her "stomach."

On examination she has a low-grade fever and is jaundiced. Examination of her abdomen reveals a palpable, tender mass in her right upper quadrant. Her labs reveal an elevated amylase and lipase. A right-upper quadrant ultrasound reveals no evidence of stones and a normal sized gallbladder. The common bile duct is 1 cm in diameter.

An ERCP is performed to evaluate for a potentially impacted stone. There is no stone found, but an abnormality of the biliary tree is evident (Figure 37-1).

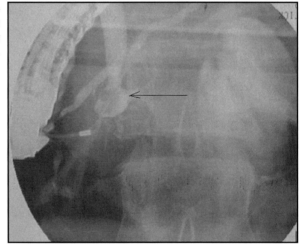

Figure 37-1. ERCP in 23-year-old with recurrent pancreatitis. (Used with permission from Ginsberg G, Ahmad N, eds. *The Clinician's Guide to Pancreaticobiliary Disorders.* Thorofare, NJ: SLACK Incorporated; 2006.)

▶ **What is the diagnosis?**

▶ **What is the most feared long-term complication of this diagnosis?**

▶ **How should this be treated?**

Vignette 37: Answer

This is a type III choledochal cyst, also known as a choledochocele. Choledochal cysts are segmental dilatations of the biliary tree that can lead to a range of complications, including strictures, recurrent pancreatitis, and malignant transformation to cholangiocarcinoma—the most feared consequence.

Choledochal cysts are congenital. They are categorized according to several different complex taxonomies. To keep it simple, just remember that Type I cysts are diffuse enlargements of the common bile duct, Type II cysts are diverticula of the common bile duct, Type III cysts are dilatations of the intraduodenal portion of the common bile duct (ie, a "choledochocele"), Type IV cysts are multiple intra- and extrahepatic bile duct cysts, and Type V cysts are diffuse intrahepatic cysts—like with Caroli's Disease. Type V cysts are not typically the subject of an adult Board examination (more for pediatrics), so concentrate on Types I through IV instead—and really types I through III in particular. I always had trouble remembering which was which, so I came up with a simple memory crutch when I was a fellow (Figure 37-2).

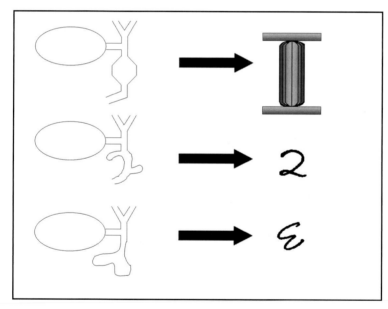

Figure 37-2. Stylized depictions of Types I through III choledochal cysts.

No doubt this is a bit contrived, but here is how it works: when you think of a Type I cyst, picture a Roman column sitting on a floor and supporting a ceiling, like in Figure 37-2. That is meant to depict a Roman numeral "I," for Type I. Now picture the column as having a taper at the top and bottom—a sort of "fusiform" shape like in Figure 37-2. This memory crutch will remind you that Type I cysts are fusiform dilatations of the common bile duct. For Type II cysts, think of the number "2." You can see how I have drawn the stylized depiction of Type II cysts to look like the number "2" is embedded in the common bile duct. The projections off the "2" make little diverticula along the common bile duct. It should be pretty self-evident as you study Figure 37-2. Finally, Type III cysts are bulging dilatations at the end of the bile duct as it enters the duodenum. I picture the number "3" flipped horizontally, as shown in Figure 37-2. You might have to use your imagination on this one, but the flipped "3" sort of depicts 2 bulges on either side of an umbilicated sphincter. Maybe just crazy and contrived enough to actually remember.

Whatever the Type, choledochal cysts are uncommon and usually present in childhood. However, they can go undetected into early adulthood, and are even diagnosed much later in life in rare occasions. There is much debate and uncertainty about how or why these form, so I'll leave that discussion for the textbooks.

What you should know is that there is a classic clinical triad associated with these cysts, including jaundice, abdominal pain, and a palpable abdominal mass from the cyst itself (although this full triad is often incomplete in adults). All choledochal cysts have malignant potential, and up to 30% of adult patients with bile duct cysts ultimately develop cholangiocarcinoma. The risk appears highest with Type I and II cysts, and lowest with Type III cysts (choledochoceles). Because the risk with Type I and II cysts is substantial, it is uniformly recommended to remove these cysts surgically. The management of Type III cysts is more controversial, since some series indicate a malignant transformation risk as low as 1% to 10%. Many authorities recommend endoscopic sphincterotomy as first-line therapy for symptomatic choledochoceles, reserving surgery for patients failing sphincterotomy or for those with recurrent complications (eg, pancreatitis).

On a Board exam, if there is a Type I or II cyst, then surgery is warranted. If there is a Type III lesion, then sphincterotomy is generally recommended, assuming there are no substantial complications (eg, recurrent pancreatitis, strictures, dysplasia on brushings, etc). If there are any alarming features, then surgery remains a reasonable option given the risk of recurrent cholangitis, pancreatitis, and cancer itself.

Why might this be tested? Remember that pancreaticobiliary accounts for 18% of the GI Board exam, so it is just a matter of time before you run into this stuff. This condition is eminently "testable" because these lesions are premalignant, and the examiners are always interested in making sure you don't blow off lesions that can turn into cancer. The same logic applies to gallbladder polyps (see Vignette 28).

Here's the Point!

Young Patient + Jaundice + Abdominal Pain + RUQ Palpable Mass = Choledochal Cyst

>> Surgery if Type I or Type II – Possible sphincterotomy for Type III <<

Vignette 38: Variceal Bleed with Eosinophilia

A 40-year-old recent immigrant from Thailand presents with acute upper GI hemorrhage. He undergoes urgent upper endoscopy that reveals multiple esophageal varices. Hemostasis is achieved with banding. On further investigation you find that he has no known history of cirrhosis. He reports drinking only socially, and never in excess. He has no history of viral hepatitis.

Physical exam reveals hepatomegaly and a markedly enlarged spleen. There are no stigmata of chronic liver disease. Laboratories are notable for eosinophilia and thrombocytopenia. Liver function tests, including albumin, INR, and bilirubin, are all normal. The transaminases are both mildly elevated (2x ULN). A liver biopsy is performed that reveals portal fibrosis with granuloma formation.

▶ *What is this?*

▶ *How is this treated?*

Vignette 38: Answer

This is schistosomiasis with resulting portal hypertension. Although not commonly diagnosed in the United States, schistosomiasis is one of the most common causes of portal hypertension worldwide. The lifecycle of this parasite is somewhat complex and beyond the scope of this limited discussion, but ultimately the eggs pass into the portal circulation in humans and get trapped in the portal venules.

This leads to a characteristic portal fibrosis and granulomas on liver biopsy with resulting portal hypertension. The portal hypertension can be severe, and typically presents with hepatomegaly, striking splenomegaly, hypersplenism (with thrombocytopenia), and variceal hemorrhage. An important clue is that liver function is invariably preserved, so true liver function tests (eg, bilirubin, INR, albumin) are typically normal. Because of the preserved synthetic function, patients with schistosomiasis-related variceal hemorrhage tolerate their bleeds better than patients with cirrhosis-related variceal bleeds. Treatment is with praziquantel.

Why might this be tested? It seems like most exams in medicine—be it GI or otherwise—invariably include one or more questions about tropical infections and infections from developing countries. This condition is relevant for the Boards not only because it meets this criterion, but also because it is extremely prevalent worldwide—not just a mere curiosity. Also, there are so many pathognomonic characteristics of this condition that it is low hanging fruit for exam questions.

Here's the Point!

Portal Hypertension + Eosinophilia + Normal Liver Function Tests + Large Spleen = Schistosomiasis

Vignette 39: GI Bleeding after Liver Biopsy

A 54-year-old man with chronic hepatitis C undergoes liver biopsy for pretreatment staging. The biopsy requires 2 passes to obtain a satisfactory core sample. The patient tolerates the procedure well and is stable during the postprocedural observation period. The following morning he awakes with abdominal discomfort and right flank pain, and subsequently passes 3 black, loose stools.

He presents to the emergency department, where he is found to have orthostatic vital signs and is started on IV fluids. A nasogastric lavage reveals clear, nonbilious output. There are no stigmata of chronic liver disease. There is an ecchymosis at the site of the liver biopsy in the right flank. Rectal examination confirms melenic stools. There is no previous history of GI bleeding. He does not use aspirin or nonsteroidal anti-inflammatory drugs. Relevant labs include: INR=1.0; Platelets=220; Hemoglobin=12.8; Albumin=3.9; AST=58; ALT=70.

▸ *What is the most likely diagnosis?*

▸ *How is this treated?*

Vignette 39: Answer

This is hemobilia resulting from a complicated percutaneous liver biopsy. Although flank pain is the most common complication of liver biopsy, occurring in around 30% of patients, bleeding is the most common serious complication of the procedure, occurring in 0.3% of cases.

The most common type of bleeding is from a liver laceration, which typically leads to intraperitoneal bleeding, or at least bleeding within the capsule of the liver. However, bleeding can track into the biliary system, as happened in this case, and feed into the hepatic ducts, common bile duct, and finally into the duodenum. The melena suggests a communication between the liver and the gastrointestinal lumen—not just bleeding into the capsule or peritoneum.

Risk factors for bleeding include multiple passes (required 2 in this case), increasing patient age, the type of needle used (cutting needles may be higher risk than suction needles), underlying hepatic malignancy, and hepatic amyloidosis (see Vignette 2 for more on amyloid). Significant thrombocytopenia, which was not present here, is an important and powerful risk factor for bleeding after liver biopsy, and is a contraindication to the percutaneous approach. Transjugular biopsy should be used in the setting of low platelets.

Although some providers might do an endoscopy first, that is generally a waste of time in suspected hemobilia. In this case, at least, the pretest likelihood of hemobilia is so high that endoscopy is not necessary to make the diagnosis. Moreover, endoscopy cannot provide definitive hemostasis of any kind—only angiography with selective embolization of the culprit artery can stop this bleeding. If that fails, then surgical ligation may be necessary.

Although not directly germane to this vignette, it is worth reviewing how to interpret nasogastric lavage results. In this instance the lavage yielded nonbilious, clear fluid. Yet the patient indeed had active bleeding into the duodenum. This emphasizes that nasogastric lavage, although very specific, is not highly sensitive—particularly for distal foregut bleeding. Figure 39-1 provides a simple algorithm for interpreting nasogastric lavage results. If the lavage reveals frank blood, then naturally the patient is actively bleeding. If there is no frank blood, then the next step is to establish whether the output is bilious or not bilious.

Bilious output is typically described as greenish-yellow. If the output is clear and bilious, then there is a <5% chance of ongoing bleeding from the foregut, including the duodenum. Bilious output implies that either the nasogastric tube has passed the pylorus and is sitting in the duodenum, or else it is still in the stomach but the pylorus is partly incompetent, thus allowing duodenal contents to reflux into the stomach. If the output is clear but not bilious—as occurred here—then there is still up to a 15% chance of ongoing foregut bleeding (ie, from a duodenal ulcer or, in this case, hemobilia). Despite the apparent certainty of this algorithmic approach, it is important to note that routine nasogastric lavage remains somewhat controversial in the literature, and that the true sensitivity, specificity, and even inter- and intraobserver reliability for this test remains variable.

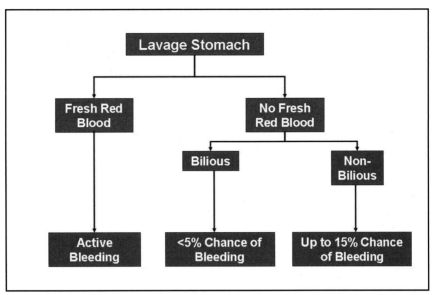

Figure 39-1. Interpreting nasogastric lavage in setting of suspected upper GI hemorrhage.

Why might this be tested? As the worldwide prevalence of liver disease continues to rise, there will be an increasing use of liver biopsy. So it is critical to be familiar with the common complications of this procedure, and bleeding is amongst the most common. Also, it is important to understand that hemobilia, or "bleeding from beyond," is not treated with endoscopic therapy. Whether hemobilia is from "hemosuccus pancreaticus" (bleeding from the pancreatic duct), cholangiocarcinoma, liver cancer, or a complication of liver biopsy, they all need angiography as the first line test to identify and treat acute hemorrhage.

Here's the Point #1

GI Bleeding after Liver Biopsy = Think Hemobilia

Here's the Point #2

Clear but non-bilious nasogastric aspirate does not rule out a duodenal source of bleeding. Clear but bilious fluid is much more specific.

Vignette 40: Abdominal Cramping in a Young Woman

A 22-year-old woman presents for evaluation of recurrent left-sided lower abdominal cramping. The symptoms first began 10 years ago and have occurred monthly ever since. She describes the cramping as a "tightness" that sometimes develops into a "gas pain" that only improves by taking nonsteroidal anti-inflammatory drugs. The symptoms usually last 3 to 5 days and always improve. There are no symptoms between bouts.

When present, the cramping does not improve with BMs, and is not associated with food intake. There is no associated diarrhea, constipation, or rectal bleeding. Her weight has remained stable for years, and she has an appropriate appetite. She has no fevers, chills, or sweats.

Upon hearing about lower abdominal symptoms, her primary care physician ordered a barium enema, which was normal. The exam was conducted between bouts. A follow-up barium enema was performed during a bout of abdominal discomfort, and it revealed a 2- to 3-cm nodule in her sigmoid colon.

She was then referred to you for a colonoscopy, which you subsequently performed during a symptom bout. The colonoscopy confirmed a roughly 3-cm subepithelial nodule. The remainder of the colon was unremarkable. Epithelial biopsies were unremarkable. A follow-up EUS was performed between bouts, and was normal—the nodule was not seen.

▶ **What is the most likely diagnosis?**

▶ **To whom should you refer the patient next, and for what test?**

Vignette 40: Answer

This is intestinal endometriosis. We often do not think about endometriosis as a cause of abdominal pain, in contrast to pelvic pain. But endometriosis is probably more common than we think in our GI practices, so it is important to be aware of the GI manifestations of this prevalent condition. Although endometriosis typically affects the pelvis, up to one-third of patients with active endometriosis have intestinal involvement.

When the GI tract is affected, endometriosis is typically limited to the serosa, and does not usually penetrate into the lumen. However, when the lesions swell during cyclic peaks, they can appear as subepithelial nodules, both on radiographic and endoscopic examinations. In some cases the nodules can become so large, either just before or during menses, that they can obstruct the lumen. In rare instances the lesions can erode into the lumen and cause bleeding. Because of its predilection for younger patients, its common involvement of the rectum, and its ability to create "stricture-like" obstructions, colonic endometriosis is often mistaken for Crohn's Disease. Don't be fooled.

In this case the clues are the cyclical pattern, the onset at around the time of puberty, the lack of association with food intake or abnormalities in stool frequency or form (arguing against IBS), and the waxing and waning subepithelial nodule. The next step would be to refer this patient to a gynecologist. The definitive diagnostic test is laparoscopy.

Why might this be tested? Because it is easy for GI doctors to forget about gynecological disorders, despite the fact that these disorders often overlap with GI conditions. Endometriosis is common, and GI involvement is also common. So this is not a mere curiosity—it is something each of us has probably seen and missed sometime during our career.

Here's the Point!

Premenopausal Women with Cyclical Abdominal Pain = Think GI Endometriosis

Vignette 41: Neutropenia and Bowel Trouble

You are called to evaluate an inpatient with new-onset abdominal pain. The patient is a 56-year-old man who was admitted 1 week ago to receive chemotherapy for chronic lymphocytic leukemia. He developed fevers, watery bloody diarrhea, and right lower quadrant abdominal pain within 2 days of the absolute neutrophil count falling below 100.

On examination he has no discernible bowel sounds. His abdomen is slightly distended and tympanitic. There is marked rebound tenderness, most notably in the right lower quadrant of his abdomen. Rectal examination is deferred due to his neutropenia, but examination of a recently passed BM reveals liquid brown stool with maroon blood. A CT scan of the abdomen is performed and reveals thickening of the cecum and ascending colon.

▶ **What is the diagnosis?**

▶ **Is colonoscopy indicated?**

Vignette 41: Answer

This is typhlitis, or neutropenic enterocolitis, affecting the cecum and terminal ileum. Typhlitis is intestinal inflammation that occurs in the setting of severe neutropenia—most commonly during treatment of leukemia or lymphoma. It has also been described in AIDS.

Typhlitis most commonly affects the cecum, appendix, or terminal ileum. The etiology remains unclear, but is thought to involve unchecked inflammation with resulting necrosis, possibly from underlying infections in the setting of severe immunocompromise (eg, neutropenia, AIDS). It is unclear whether the infection comes first, or if infection is a secondary consequence of an initial event that disrupts the barrier function of the bowel. The cecum is particularly vulnerable because its thin wall is susceptible to perforation in the setting of inflammation and necrosis. Because typhlitis is a necrotizing process, the main risk is development of cecal distention, ischemia, ulceration, and ultimately perforation of the bowel.

Patients typically complain of abdominal pain, nausea, vomiting, and watery diarrhea that can be bloody. Examination can range from minor tenderness in the right lower quadrant to an acute abdomen with ileus—eg, absent bowel sounds, guarding, and rigidity. The differential diagnosis includes infectious colitis (especially *C. difficile* colitis, which can sometimes affect the cecum in particular), appendicitis, and ischemic colitis, among others. The diagnosis is often raised after a CT scan reveals a thickened cecum and ascending colon, as in this case.

Stool studies must be sent for culture and *C. difficile* toxins prior to confirming typhlitis as the etiology. Colonoscopy, when performed, may reveal erythema and mucosal friability in the cecum and ascending colon. However, colonoscopy is rarely performed and generally ill-advised since these patients are neutropenic (even a rectal examination is typically contraindicated) and because the risk of perforation is high.

Treatment of typhlitis typically starts with bowel rest, intravenous fluids, and broad spectrum antibiotics (including fungal coverage) to help avoid superinfection. Because typhlitis tends to occur in severely ill and neutropenic patients, surgical intervention is rarely, if ever, the first line therapy. Surgery is generally reserved for patients with outright perforation, or those with severe persistent typhlitis despite conservative therapy. Surgery carries a substantial risk of mortality. The overall mortality rate of typhlitis is 50%.

Why might this be tested? Although typhlitis is relatively uncommon, it definitely happens, so it is important to know about this condition. In particular, you need to know that colonoscopy carries a very high risk for perforation. So this is one of those topics where the examiners may want to confirm you don't do something foolish, like start scoping just because there is bloody diarrhea. In this case, scoping could potentially cause more harm than good.

Here's the Point!

Neutropenia + Right Lower Quadrant Abdominal Pain +
Thickened Cecum on CT = Typhlitis
>> Colonoscopy generally contraindicated! <<

Vignette 42: Recurrent Abdominal Pain and Vomiting

A 38-year-old woman presents with recurrent epigastric pain, nausea, and vomiting. These symptoms have occurred on-and-off for most of her life, but have become more frequent and severe over the last year. She underwent upper endoscopy, which revealed a normal esophagus and stomach, but an abnormally narrow second part of the duodenum. There were no mucosal-based lesions. Instead, it appeared as if there was an extrinsic compression of the lumen.

A follow-up CT scan (Figure 42-1) reveals an enlarged head of the pancreas, but no focal mass.

Figure 42-1. Results of patient's cholangiogram. (Courtesy of James Farrell, MD, David Geffen School of Medicine at UCLA.)

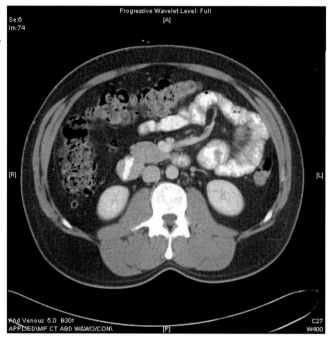

▶ **What is the diagnosis?**

▶ **What is the next diagnostic step to confirm the diagnosis?**

Vignette 42: Answer

This is an annular pancreas. Annular pancreas is a congenital anomaly resulting from failure of the left ventral bud of the pancreas to fully rotate during embryological development. In reality, the exact mechanism of annular pancreas remains somewhat controversial, but do not worry about that for Boards. The bottom line is that the pancreas is wrapped around the second part of the duodenum, and this leads to an extrinsic compression. When severe, it can cause an almost complete foregut obstruction and is diagnosed at birth, where it presents with a "double bubble" sign on radiography. However, most patients remain asymptomatic and have partial, if any, duodenal obstruction.

Adults can occasionally develop new symptoms after many years of living with an annular pancreas. Typical symptoms include postprandial fullness, nausea, and vomiting. A CT scan may reveal an enlarged head of the pancreas without a focal mass (see Figure 42-1). The definitive diagnosis relies on ERCP with cholangiography, which reveals a "ring like" pancreatic duct surrounding the duodenum in addition to the usual pancreatic duct.

Treatment typically involves surgical bypass of the encircling pancreas. This strategy is preferred over surgical division of the annual ring given the attendant complications of pancreas surgery in general. This is distinguished from pancreas divisum—the most common congenital anomaly of the pancreas—which is marked by incomplete fusion of the dorsal and ventral buds. Whereas the cholangiograms in annular pancreas reveal an encircling aberrant pancreatic duct, the cholangiograms in pancreas divisum reveal 2 separate drainage systems without an encircling structure.

Why might this be tested? Cholangiograms often appear on the Board exam, and this is one of the classics. Other classics include pancreas divisum (see above), type III choledochal cysts (see Vignette 37), the "string of lakes" in sclerosing cholangitis, Mirizzi's Syndrome (stone in the cystic duct leading to compression of the common bile duct and mimicking cancer), "double duct" sign of pancreatic head cancer, and pancreaticopleural fistulae, among several others.

Here's the Point!

Early Satiety + Extrinsic Compression of Second Duodenum + Enlarged Pancreatic Head on CT Without Focal Mass = Annular Pancreas… Do ERCP, which will reveal ductal ring.

Vignette 43: Anasarca and Hepatitis C

You are called to consult on an inpatient with hepatitis C. The patient is a 54-year-old man with genotype 1 hepatitis C, contracted through intravenous drug use 2 decades ago, who has no previous evidence of cirrhosis, fibrosis, or any other sequelae of chronic hepatitis C infection.

He was in his usual state of health until 2 weeks prior to admission, when he developed ankle edema that quickly spread up his legs. Within 1 week, he developed severe swelling in his legs, abdomen, and scrotum, along with severe upper abdominal pain. Two days prior to admission he developed a rash across his thighs and arms.

Upon admission, he was found to have 3+ pitting edema in the lower extremity and flanks. There was no evidence of ascites, nor any stigmata of chronic liver disease. His skin revealed palpable purpuric lesions over the thighs and forearms. Abnormal labs include: creatinine=3.2; albumin=1.8; 24 hour urine protein=5 g; AST=55; ALT=62; ALP=50; total bilirubin=1.3; INR=1.0. Complement levels are low.

▶ *What is the diagnosis?*

▶ *Is treatment of hepatitis C indicated at this time?*

Vignette 43: Answer

This is an acute case of mixed cryoglobulinemia. Hepatitis C is the most common cause of cryoglobulinemia. Up to half of patients with hepatitis C have detectable cryoglobulins, although most patients do not suffer consequences from these circulating, temperature sensitive immunoglobulins.

Cryoglobulins precipitate out of solution at temperatures below 37°C, and can redissolve when rewarmed. Of course, this is relevant because cryoglobulins can precipitate out of solution while in blood vessels, leading to a wide range of seemingly disparate consequences, including arthritis, glomerulonephritis, neuropathy, abdominal pain from bowel vasculitis, and a leukocytoclastic vasculitis, which typically presents with palpable purpura in the lower extremities. Cryoglobulinemia is also marked by low C4 levels and a positive rheumatoid factor.

As an aside, if you lowered the age of this patient to 16 years old, added some abdominal pain, and removed the hepatitis C, then Henoch-Schonlein Purpura would be the leading diagnosis. It too can present with low C4 levels, abdominal pain, and a leukocytoclastic vasculitis. Keep that diagnosis in mind on the Boards, because even though Henoch-Schonlein Purpura is most common in kids, around 10% of the time it affects adults.

This is a real case of a consult to our inpatient GI service while I was attending. We were asked to consider treatment for hepatitis C in the setting of likely acute cryoglobulinemia. We opted to not treat, primarily because treatment of hepatitis C has little role in the acute setting of acute cryoglobulinemia, particularly when there is such severe renal disease as to cause nephrotic syndrome. Genotype 1 hepatitis C takes 12 months to treat, and has a 30% to 50% treatment success rate. So acute treatment has little role here.

The patient instead received plasmapheresis, and subsequently improved dramatically. But treatment of hepatitis C is still warranted in the long run, and must be considered once the acute illness has passed and the patient is stabilized and prepared for long-term treatment.

Why might this be tested? This is a classic, because it is one of those diagnoses that affects nearly every organ system, and has a nice, stereotyped presentation. In this vignette, which is a real case, the diagnosis was actually in doubt for a few days. The dermatology service was called to evaluate the skin rash, and diagnosed "folliculitis."

A renal biopsy was commissioned to further investigate the etiology of the nephrotic syndrome. Our service was called because of a history of hepatitis C. The primary team wondered whether treatment was indicated given the association with cryoglobulinemia—a diagnosis they had been considering but fell lower on the list after dermatology called "folliculitis."

We went to the bedside, and respectfully disagreed with the skin diagnosis. We were convinced the lesions were indeed a leukocytoclastic vasculitis, and that very few things other than cryoglobulinemia could cause abrupt nephrotic syndrome, abdominal pain, low complement levels, and a skin rash in the setting of hepatitis C. So, this diagnosis is just a classic, and is bound to show up either on a Board exam, in real life, or in both settings.

Here's the Point #1

Hepatitis C + Positive Rheumatoid Factor + Low Complement + Lower Extremity Purpuric Rash + Paresthesias + Renal Disease = Mixed Cryoglobulinemia

Here's the Point #2

Young Adult + Abdominal Pain + Low Complement + Purpuric Rash on Thighs = Henoch-Schonlein Purpura

Vignette 44: Bumps on Face and Bowels

A 59-year-old woman is referred for colon cancer screening. She has a family history of "colon polyps" of unknown histology in her older sister and mother. On examination you notice small papules on her hands, feet, and face. There is "cobblestoning" on her tongue. Colonoscopy reveals multiple polyps throughout her large bowel. Subsequent histology indicates that the polyps are hamartomatous.

▸ **What is the diagnosis?**

▸ **What are the bumps?**

▸ **Is this inherited?**

Vignette 44: Answer

This is Cowden's Syndrome. Cowden's Syndrome is an autosomal dominant disorder arising from a germline mutation in PTEN, a tumor suppressor gene. The PTEN mutation is identified in 80% of probands with Cowden's Syndrome.

Cowden's is characterized by hamartomatous tumors throughout the GI tract. It is unknown whether Cowden's increases the risk of colon cancer. However, the disorder is associated with an increased risk of breast, thyroid, and endometrial neoplasia. The breast cancer may be bilateral, and the thyroid involvement is typically papillary cancer. Mucocutaneous lesions are found in 90% of patients, most notably trichilemmomas—the "bumps" on the face, hands, and feet in this vignette. The mucosal lesions can coalesce in the buccal mucosa and lead to a cobblestone-like pattern in 40% of patients.

Because the risk of colorectal cancer remains unclear, there are no explicit guidelines on whether, or how, to perform surveillance colonoscopy—currently these patients should receive age-appropriate colorectal cancer screening. Surveillance for other neoplasms (ie, breast, thyroid, endometrial) must occur in all patients with Cowden's.

Why might this be tested? Examiners love to test on hereditary syndromes in general, and hereditary polyp syndromes in particular (see Vignettes 151-156 for more on these syndromes). Cowden's syndrome has some stereotyped features and "buzzwords" that lend themselves to a Board question—ie, "trichilemmomas," "cobblestoning," etc. And, as always, the Boards love questions that test knowledge about dermatological manifestations of GI diseases.

Here's the Point!

Hamartomas + Cobblestoned Tongue + Bumps on Face = Cowden's Syndrome

Vignettes 45-50: Isolated Elevated ALP/GGT

You will commonly come across patients who have an elevated ALP, but who have a normal AST, ALT, bilirubin, albumin, LDH, and INR. These patients have "isolated elevated ALP." There is a relatively short differential diagnosis for this biochemical profile. In some instances the GGT is concurrently elevated (let's call that "isolated elevated ALP/GGT"), and in some instances it is not. Name the diagnosis for each "mini-vignette," below:

High ALP, normal AST, ALT, bilirubin, albumin, LDH, INR, and....

45. Fever, weight loss, costovertebral angle tenderness, microscopic hematuria, and normal GGT.

46. Headache, visual changes, markedly elevated ESR, and concurrently elevated GGT.

47. Weight loss, microcytic anemia, fecal occult positive stool, concurrently elevated GGT.

48. Flushing with alcohol ingestion + Intermittent hypotension + Darier's Sign + Abdominal pain + Malabsorption + Hepatosplenomegaly + Concurrently elevated GGT (this has to be something!).

49. Angioid streaks in eyes, normal GGT.

50. Morning stiffness in hands, subcutaneous nodules along forearms, concurrently elevated GGT.

Vignettes 45-50: Answers

45. This is renal cell carcinoma. Renal cell is called "the internist's tumor" because it can present with many disparate clinical features. The alkaline phosphatase (ALP) can be elevated with a renal cell carcinoma, but the gamma-glutamyl transpeptidase (GGT) should not be elevated.

46. This is temporal arteritis. Here is a true story: our inpatient GI consult service was called to place a PEG tube in a 72-year-old man with "aspiration pneumonia and dementia."

In reviewing the laboratories, we found that his GGT was elevated at around 250, and his ALP was elevated as well. The AST, ALT, TB, albumin, and INR were all unremarkable, and he had no stigmata of chronic liver disease. On exam we noticed that his temporal arteries were thick bilaterally and "cord-like." Suspecting temporal arteritis, we asked his daughter (who was at the bedside) about headaches, visual changes, and jaw claudication. She explained that he recently had monocular visual deficits, and that he had increasingly complained of headaches. We ordered an ESR and it came back at 122. He was started on steroids.

One point here is that a GI consult should be a medicine consult—even if only done for a PEG placement. The entire symptom complex could have been explained by temporal arteritis alone, including the pulmonary symptoms (can present with a Churg-Strauss like vasculitis picture in the lungs), fevers, and mental status changes. So a PEG would not have addressed those issues. The other point is to simply remember that an isolated elevated ALP or GGT in an old person should make you think about temporal arteritis, particularly if there have been headaches or visual changes. This is one condition that must be treated quickly or else serious sequelae will result—namely blindness.

47. This is colon cancer with metastasis to the liver. Space-filling lesions in the liver can lead to isolated elevated ALP/GGT. This occurs because there is compression of the bile canniculi (leading to spillage of ALP and GGT), but the liver parenchyma and overall liver function is usually preserved. So the "liver function tests" (ie, bilirubin, albumin, INR) and other liver tests (ie, AST, ALT) are usually normal, or at least not as elevated as the ALP/GGT. Typical space-forming lesions in the liver include intrinsic tumors, metastatic tumors, abscesses, cysts, sarcoid, and amyloid, among others. In this case the microcytic anemia and occult blood positivity point to colon cancer with likely metastasis to the liver—the most common metastatic target of colorectal cancer.

48. This is systemic mastocytosis. This condition is an examiner favorite because it presents in so many different ways and affects nearly every major organ system. Mastocytosis is a systemic disorder characterized by mast cell infiltration of several systems, including lymph nodes, spleen, skin, bone marrow, CNS, GI tract, and the liver. The high ALP occurs because of diffuse infiltration of the liver with mast cells. The mast cell infiltrates secrete histamine, which, in turn, can lead to hypersecretion of acid in the stomach with peptic ulcers and acid reflux disease. This is a rare hyper-acidic syndrome that can be treated as effectively with a histamine-2 receptor blocker as with a PPI. Mastocytosis can lead to periodic flushing (particularly with alcohol ingestion), abdominal pain, diarrhea with malabsorption, paresthesias, low blood pressure (histamine mediated), and just about anything else. A fun fact is that it is associated with Darier's sign, which is visible urticaria from scratching the skin.

49. This is Paget's Disease. Paget's can lead to ALP elevation through its effects on bone. The GGT will be normal. "Angioid streaks" in the retina are characteristic of only a few conditions, one of them being Paget's Disease. The other condition with GI relevance and angioid streaks is pseudoxanthoma elasticum (PXE)—a condition marked by abnormal collagen deposition and upper GI bleeding (see Vignette 15 for details).

50. This is RA. RA can affect virtually every organ system in the body. Not uncommonly, RA can affect the liver, sometimes presenting only with an isolated elevated GGT or ALP. Recall that Felty's Syndrome is the unique combination of RA, splenomegaly, and neutropenia. This is relevant, because Felty's Syndrome can sometimes present with nodular regenerative hyperplasia (NRH) of the liver (see Vignette 116 for more details on NRH) and even portal hypertension. RA is also associated with chronic hepatitis, amyloidosis (can infiltrate the liver and lead to elevated ALP/GGT), and rarely primary biliary cirrhosis (can also present with high ALP/GGT).

Vignette 51: Recurrent Vomiting

A 23-year-old man presents with intermittent vomiting for the last 2 years. The symptoms first began while he was serving in Iraq, where he participated in active combat duties. During that time he experienced spells of vomiting on several occasions. The other members of his troop did not suffer from vomiting.

The episodes continued after discharge. Typically he is fine and does not suffer from any GI symptoms. After months of feeling well, he develops abrupt nausea, followed by vomiting within hours. The vomiting continues for weeks at a time, often to the point of presenting to the emergency department for antiemetics and intravenous hydration. The bouts always pass spontaneously, and he returns to his usual state of good health.

He is unable to identify specific triggers. The bouts can begin any time of day. He does not suffer from undue anxiety or depression. He does not suffer from migraine headaches. He uses marijuana intermittently.

▶ **What is the most likely diagnosis?**

▶ **Does this have anything to do with marijuana?**

Vignette 51: Answer

This is cyclical vomiting syndrome (CVS). CVS is a rare and often devastating condition marked by intermittent and prolonged bouts of seemingly unstoppable vomiting, separated by periods of complete calm—thus its "cyclical" nature. CVS was first recognized in children, but has been increasingly acknowledged as a condition that can affect adults. In children it is more common in boys, but in adults it affects both sexes equally.

Nobody knows what causes CVS. It is classified as a functional gastrointestinal disorder (FGID). Because many FGIDs are associated with chronic stress and anxiety (eg, IBS, functional abdominal pain syndrome, etc), some believe that CVS can be triggered by stressful events (in this case active combat exposure). However, others have found genetic abnormalities in patients with CVS, and some even believe that CVS results from inheritance of abnormal DNA sequence variations from maternal mitochrondria.

I'll leave the details to other sources—particularly since nobody knows the answer, so pathogenesis is unlikely to be on a Board exam. But diagnosing CVS is certainly Board eligible material. The usual trap is to diagnose gastroenteritis or other common GI conditions (GERD, etc). Given the lack of any obvious infectious exposures, coupled with the cyclical nature of the symptoms, CVS must be considered high in the differential diagnosis for this patient.

The use of marijuana is relevant, because some believe that marijuana can trigger bouts of vomiting, and may even underlie CVS in some patients. It is important to tell patients about this relationship, and to encourage them to discontinue marijuana. Because CVS can be so life altering, most patients are all too willing to stop marijuana if they think there is any chance it is related to their symptoms.

The treatment of CVS bouts is nonspecific. Some use antimigraine medications like triptans. Others use anxiolytics like benzodiazepines. Bottom line is that the treatment is variable and not evidence-based—namely because CVS is so rare that proper randomized trials have been hard to complete.

Why might this be tested? CVS is rare but it does happen, so you should know about it. One reason examiners may like this is because they want to establish whether you'll take the obvious yet incorrect route of diagnosing viral gastroenteritis in someone who has a totally different condition. CVS patients are often undiagnosed for years, and may ultimately receive a "psychological" label or undergo a range of diagnostic tests that are unrevealing (although I for one would certainly consider endoscopy, basic laboratory tests, etc).

Here's the Point!

> **Recurrent vomiting with normal bouts in between + marijuana = think CVS**

Vignette 52: Elevated Transaminases in HIV

A 46-year-old man with AIDS, CD4<200, develops jaundice and progressive weight loss along with fevers, nausea, anorexia, and abdominal pain. This occurred after developing cutaneous papules on his hands marked by central umbilications.

Examination reveals bacillary angiomatosis lesions on his skin and an enlarged, tender liver. Relevant laboratories include: AST=112; ALT=154; ALP=320; Total Bilirubin=1.2. A CT scan of the abdomen reveals abdominal lymphadenopathy and an enlarged, diffusely heterogeneous liver.

▶ *What is the most likely diagnosis?*

▶ *What will a liver biopsy reveal?*

▶ *How is this treated?*

Vignette 52: Answer

This is peliosis hepatis from underlying *Bartonella henselae*. Peliosis hepatis is a rare liver disorder marked by multiple blood-filled cystic spaces throughout the parenchyma (not to be confused with veno occlusive disease, as described in Vignette 36). The cysts of peliosis hepatis do not have endothelial lining, but instead communicate directly with the hepatic sinusoidal system.

Peliosis is associated with a range of conditions, including HIV, where it is most commonly a consequence of *Bartonella* infection. The presence of comorbid bacillary angiomatosis—a result of *Bartonella henselae*—is highly suggestive of peliosis hepatis from *Bartonella*. The condition is also found in nonimmunosuppressed patients, who are also eligible to develop *Bartonella henselae* infections.

Peliosis has been described in users of anabolic steroids, along with a long list of other medications, including azathioprine, oral contraceptives, vitamin A, and hydroxyurea, among others. Rather than memorize this tedious list, you should focus on remembering anabolic steroids and HIV as the most common and important associations.

Peliosis usually presents with fever, weight loss, and jaundice in the setting of an enlarged liver. Because peliosis involves cystic lesions in the liver, the ALP and GGT are elevated, and out of proportion to the AST and ALT (which are also usually elevated). The bilirubin is characteristically normal or near normal. CT scans will show an enlarged and heterogenous liver, and may also reveal a large spleen and abdominal lymphadenopathy. Treatment is with erythromycin 2 g daily.

Why might this be tested? HIV-related complications are common on Board examinations, and this is one of the rare but classic liver manifestations of HIV.

Here's the Point!

AIDS + Jaundice + Cystic Blood-Filled Spaces on Liver Biopsy =
Peliosis Hepatis

Vignettes 53-59: Name that Pathogen

Name the most likely pathogen for each scenario listed below:

53. Diarrhea after consuming raw shellfish in the Gulf Coast region of the United States.

54. Diarrhea after consuming chocolate milk.

55. Diarrhea after consuming reheated fried rice.

56. Bloody diarrhea after consuming undercooked beef.

57. Diarrhea while on a cruise ship.

58. Diarrhea after buying a new pet turtle.

59. Diarrhea in cirrhosis leading to sepsis and death.

Vignettes 53-59: Answers

53. This is *Vibrio*—either *V. vulinficus* or *V. parahemolyticus*. Both the *vulinficus* and *parahemolyticus* species are associated with undercooked or raw seafood, including shellfish in particular. These organisms can also infect other types of food that are contaminated with seawater. *Vibrio* species are particularly prevalent in the Gulf Coast region of the United States, and infections are most common during the summer months.

54. This is *Listeria monocytogenes*. Listeria seems to show up all over the place, because it is a robust organism whose growth is not halted by refrigeration. It is classically associated with chocolate milk, but is also found in lunch meats, cheeses, and hot dogs, among other "summertime foods." Listeria is usually a short-lived infection, but it can cause particular trouble in vulnerable subgroups, including pregnant women, the elderly, and the immunocompromised. In these patients it can lead to systemic bacteremia and severe infections, sometimes leading to mortality (or abortion in pregnant women).

55. This is *Bacillus cereus*. Most people remember this one from medical school, because it is such a classic. It is a toxin-mediated form of food poisoning, much like *S. aureus*, so it first begins with nausea and vomiting within hours of ingestion. Diarrhea comes later. This biphasic illness pattern should trigger "toxin-mediated" in your brain, and should bring *B. cereus, S. aureus,* and *Clostridium perfringens* to mind right away—the 3 big toxin-mediated forms of food poisoning.

56. This is Enterohemorrhagic *E. coli* (EHEC) serotype O157:H7. *E. coli* 0157: H7 is an important organism because it is probably the most common cause of bloody diarrhea in the United States. Classically associated with undercooked beef, EHEC can lead to hemorrhagic colitis and even hemolytic uremic syndrome (HUS) with thrombotic thrombocytopenic purpura (TTP). EHEC is often confused for ischemic colitis, so it should always be kept in mind when ischemic colitis is being considered, particularly if there has been recent exposure to culprit foods (not only undercooked beef, but also unpasteurized milk, sprouts, lettuce, and salamis). Fever is characteristically absent in this condition. Antibiotics do not provide substantial benefits during the acute phase, and might even precipitate HUS-TTP. So best not to use them. Classic exam question: dropping hemoglobin and platelets in the setting of rising creatinine, fevers, and mental status changes after using antibiotics for bloody diarrhea (antibiotic-precipitated HUS-TTP).

57. This is Norwalk virus. Norwalk virus is one of the most common causes of infectious diarrhea in adults. Norwalk is a robust organism that can survive all sorts of threats, including chlorination and other forms of disinfection. For some reason the virus seems to end up on cruise ships, and has been the subject of intermittent news reports about shipwide outbreaks of watery diarrhea. Person-to-person spread is common, so tightly packed environments (eg, cruise ship) can promote outbreaks. Like *Vibrio* species, Norwalk virus is also associated with shellfish.

58. This is *Salmonella*. There are all types of *Salmonella* infections of the GI tract, including *S. typhi, S. paratyphi, S. enteritidis,* and *S. typhimurium,* among over 1000 other species. *S. typhi* and *paratyphi* cause typhoid fever, while *S. enteritidis* and *typhimurium* cause nontyphoidal salmonellosis. All *Salmonella* species can be transmitted and carried by reptiles and turtles – the association in this vignette. Of course, the classic association is with undercooked eggs, poultry, meat, and dairy products. See Vignette 129 for more on *Salmonella*.

59. This is *Vibrio vulnificus* (again). See Vignette 53, above, for background information on *V. vulnificus*. Importantly, this organism is especially virulent in patients with chronic liver disease. It can lead to sepsis and death in patients with cirrhosis. For this reason, all patients with cirrhosis must be instructed to avoid eating, or even handling, raw seafood. Oysters, in particular, are a major culprit for disseminated infections and poor outcomes in cirrhosis.

Here's the Point #2

Diarrhea and...
Gulf Coast = *Vibrio*
Chocolate Milk = *Listeria*
Fried Rice = *B. cereus*
Hamburger = *E. coli* 0157:H7
Cruise Ship = Norwalk virus
Turtle / Reptile = *Salmonella*
Cirrhosis = *V. vulnificus*

Vignettes 60-65: Know Your Metabolites

Each row below represents a separate patient on either azathioprine or 6-mercaptopurine (a patient with Crohn's Disease, for example). In each case there is a 6-thioguanine (6-TG) and 6-methylmercaptopurine (6-MMP) level provided—either high, normal, low, or undetectable. For each case, fill in the explanation for the metabolite profile.

Vignette	6-TG Level	6-MMP Level	Diagnosis/Explanation
60	Normal	Normal	
61	Low	Low	
62	Low	High	
63	High	Low	
64	High	High	
65	Undetectable	Undetectable	

Vignettes 60-65: Answers

In order to answer these questions, we must first review the basic metabolic pathways of azathioprine (AZA) and 6-mercaptopurine (6-MP). Figure 60-1 provides an overview of the pathways.

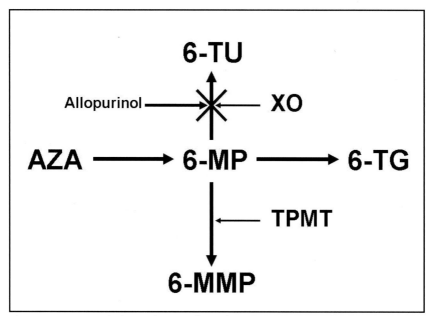

Figure 60-1. Metabolic pathway of azathioprine (AZA) and 6-mercatopurine (6MP).

AZA is nonenzymatically converted into 6-MP. In doing so, about half of AZA's therapeutic efficacy is lost. This has clinical relevance because milligram-per-milligram AZA is half as powerful as 6-MP. That is, because 6-MP is farther down the metabolic pathway, it should be dosed at about half that of AZA. The usual starting dose of 6-MP is 1.5 mg/kg/day, whereas AZA is typically started at 2.5 to 3.0 mg/kg/day. 6-MP, in turn, can be broken town into 1 of 3 byproducts.

Xanthine oxidase (XO) metabolizes 6-MP into 6-thiouric acid (6-TU), an inactive metabolic byproduct. Allopurinol can block XO, which tends to shunt 6-MP to the other 2 pathways. In patients with gout on allopurinol, it is important to remember that more toxic metabolites (namely 6-TG and 6-MMP) can be created, so dosing should be lower at first.

Thiopurine methyltransferase (TPMT) catalyzes the breakdown of 6-MP to 6-MMP, an inactive metabolite that can cause hepatotoxicity. This enzyme is important because genetic variations in TPMT have big implications in AZA/6MP dosing and toxicity. Ninety percent of the population is heterozygous for the TPMT gene—so-called high/low inheritance. In these patients, dosing of AZA/6MP can proceed according to usual algorithms.

However, around 9% to 10% of the population has a mutant genotype leading to low or absent TPMT activity—so-called low/low inheritance. These patients shunt 6-MP to 6-thioguanine (6-TG), the active metabolite that is necessary for efficacy, but that also leads to myelosuppression. The normal target is to keep 6-TG above a level of 235 in order to ensure adequate efficacy. But levels above 450 can lead to bone marrow suppression. So, patients with low/low inheritance must start with very low doses of AZA/6MP—many cannot tolerate it at all.

Finally, less than 1% of patients have the high/high inheritance, in which they have high TPMT levels and shunt most of their pathway to production of 6-MMP. These patients can have hepatotoxicity. 6-MMP levels above 5700 are typically associated with liver toxicity, and should be avoided. For what it is worth, some believe that mesalamine and sulfasalazine (ie, 5-ASA) can inhibit TPMT, thus shunting 6MP to its active metabolite 6-TG.

So, with this overview the vignettes should now make sense, as follows:

60. Therapeutic. Both levels are within normal range, suggesting therapeutic dosing of AZA/6MP.

61. Underdosed. Both levels are low, suggesting inadequate dosing.

62. High/High Inheritance of TPMT. There is too much 6-MMP, which is bad (hepatotoxic). At the same time, there is too little 6-TG, which is also bad (no efficacy). This suggests that TPMT is hyperactive, and is shunting 6MP to 6-MMP instead of T-TG. The dose may need to be raised, although it might be hard to use AZA/6MP under this circumstance.

63. Low/Low Inheritance of TPMT. There is too much 6-TG, which is bad (myelosuppressive). At the same time, there is very low 6-MMP. This combination suggests an absence or near-absence of TMPT activity, so 6MP is shunted to 6-TG. The dose needs to be lowered, although it also may be hard to use AZA/6MP in this setting.

64. Overdosed. Both levels are high, so the problem is too much drug.

65. Non-Compliant. Both levels are undetectable, so the problem is lack of drug, presumably from noncompliance with the prescribed medication.

Vignette 66: Anemia and Diarrhea

A 52-year-old man recently traveled to Puerto Rico for 3 months. He developed fatigue, malaise, and abdominal cramps 1 week after returning, followed by diarrhea and dyspepsia. He describes his stool as "oatmeal like." Relevant labs include a Hgb of 11.3 with an MCV of 103. Stool studies are negative for ova & parasites. Enteroscopy is performed. An image of the proximal jejunum is pictured in Figure 66-1.

Figure 66-1. Endoscopic appearance of proximal jejunum. (Used with permission from William Ravich, MD, Johns Hopkins University School of Medicine, Baltimore, MD.)

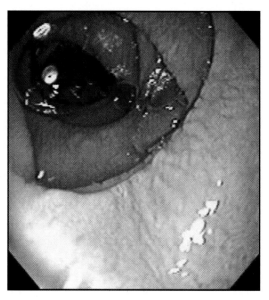

▶ **What is the most likely diagnosis?**

▶ **What abnormality is pictured in Figure 66-1?**

▶ **How is this treated?**

Vignettes 66: Answer

This is tropical sprue. Tropical sprue mimics celiac sprue because, like celiac disease, it leads to villous blunting with malabsorption. However, it is a different condition altogether.

Tropical sprue is endemic to a unique "sprue belt," including Puerto Rico, Cuba, the Dominican Republic, Haiti, India, and the Middle East. The etiology of tropical sprue remains unknown, although it is suspected to be an infectious disorder. The chronic form of tropical sprue requires 2 years of residence in an endemic region, whereas the acute form does not depend on length of stay.

Chronic tropical sprue has 3 distinct phases: Phase I includes fatigue and abdominal discomfort, but not necessarily diarrhea. Phase II includes diarrhea, dyspepsia, and overt malabsorption (typically described as "oatmeal" consistency of the stool). Phase III yields a macrocytic, megaloblastic anemia. The acute form does not progress through these neat phases, but instead presents with an accelerated clinical course with all phases nearly combined together.

Endoscopy may reveal classic sprue findings, including scalloping of the plicae circularis (as pictured in Figure 66-1), cracked mucosa, and nodularity. Histology reveals shortening of the villi, lengthening of the crypts, and a chronic inflammatory infiltrate, as with celiac sprue. Tropical sprue is usually treated with tetracycline 250 mg QID and folate 5 mg daily for 6 to 12 months.

Why might this be tested? To make sure that you can distinguish celiac sprue from tropical sprue. The treatments are quite different, so it is important that you can tell one from the other.

Here's the Point!

Diarrhea + Tropics + High MCV Anemia = Tropical Sprue

Vignette 67: Diarrhea and Nystagmus

A 46-year-old Caucasian man presents with chronic diarrhea, lethargy, hand arthralgias, and weight loss. His wife thinks his memory is fading. Examination reveals diffuse lymphadenopathy, patches of hyperpigmented skin, nystagmus, and a systolic murmur.

Upper endoscopy is performed, which reveals PAS positive "foamy macrophages" in the jejunal biopsies. The serum carotene is low. HIV is negative. Sudan stain of the stool is positive.

▶ *What is the most likely diagnosis?*

▶ *What other condition is associated with PAS positive "foamy macrophages" and diarrhea?*

▶ *How is this treated?*

Vignette 67: Answer

This is Whipple's Disease. Whipple's Disease is one of those conditions that magically affects virtually every organ system. Like amyloidosis, coccidiomycosis, lupus, sarcoid, and a slew of other "morning report favorites," Whipple's can fit a wide range of clinical presentations. In any event, Whipple's is caused by infection with the *Tropheryma whipplei*, a soil-born organism that has similarities to *Actinomycetes* species.

The hallmark finding of Whipple's Disease is "foamy macrophages" in the lamina propria of the small bowel stuffed full of the organisms, which stain positive with the PAS stain. This leads to a malabsorption syndrome, evidenced in this case by the low serum carotene and positive Sudan stain for stool fat.

Of note, MAC enteritis can present in the same manner. That is, MAC presents with diarrhea and PAS-positive "foamy macrophages" in the lamina propria of the small intestine. In this case the patient is HIV negative, making MAC enteritis much less likely. MAC can also be distinguished from Whipple's because it stains positive with the acid fast bacillus (AFB) stain, whereas *T. whipplei* stains negative for AFB. For whatever reason (maybe genetic), Whipple's is overwhelmingly more common in white men of European ancestry, so keep that in mind when reading Board vignettes where Whipple's is in the differential diagnosis.

Whipple's Disease can present in many different ways, but the most common symptoms include arthralgias, weight loss, recurrent abdominal pain, and diarrhea. The latter is from malabsorption, as noted above. The arthralgias typically affect the large joints. The weight loss can be considerable—to the point of a full blown wasting syndrome. The skin may become hyperpigmented in patches. The heart can be affected in many different ways, including a culture-negative endocarditis or pericarditis. There are also some characteristic CNS manifestations of Whipple's, including memory loss, cerebellar ataxia, and nystagmus. Interestingly, the nystagmus is no ordinary nystagmus—it is an "oculomasticatory myorhythmia" marked by contractions of the masseter muscle coupled with rhythmic eye movements. Interesting condition.

In any event, treatment is with antibiotics. Although tetracycline has been used in the past, most authorities suggest an initial course of parenteral ceftriaxone, followed by a year of twice daily trimethoprim-sulfamethozazole double-strength tablets.

Why might this be tested? Because Whipple's is, for whatever reason, a perennial exam favorite. There are just too many Board buzzwords associated with this condition (eg, PAS positive "foamy macrophages," cerebellar ataxia, oculomasticatory myorhythmia, etc) to pass it up for a Board question.

Here's the Point!

Diarrhea + Weight Loss + Abdominal Pain + Arthralgias + Acid Fast Negative, PAS Positive "Foamy Macrophages" = Whipple's Disease (not MAC)

Vignette 68: Diarrhea in Heart Failure

A 72-year-old man with New York Class III congestive heart failure is referred for diarrhea. His symptoms began 6 months ago and coincided with worsening of his heart failure. Over the last 2 months he has also experienced intermittent and progressive nausea and vomiting, along with diffuse abdominal fullness.

Examination reveals bibasilar crackles, an enlarged yet soft liver, prominent hepatojugular reflux, and shifting dullness upon abdominal percussion. There is 3+ bilateral lower extremity pitting edema. There are no stigmata of chronic liver disease.

Laboratories include: Albumin=2.4; serum carotene=8 (low); ALP=190; AST=99; ALT=85; INR=1.1. A sample of ascitic fluid from paracentesis reveals the following: Albumin=1.2; total protein=2.1; total cell count=50. A qualitative stool fat is positive. Enteroscopy reveals focal white spots scattered throughout the visualized small bowel mucosa. Biopsies are obtained and are pending.

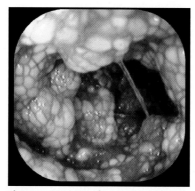

Figure 68-1. Endoscopic appearance of proximal jejunum. (Courtesy of Wilfred Weinstein, MD, David Geffen School of Medicine at UCLA.)

▶ *What is the most likely diagnosis?*

▶ *What abnormalities will be seen on the biopsies?*

▶ *Why is the albumin low?*

▶ *Why are the liver tests elevated?*

Vignette 68: Answer

This is secondary intestinal lymphangiectasia. Intestinal lymphangiectasia has primary and secondary forms. The primary form, which affects children, is an autosomal dominant condition marked by idiopathic lymphatic obstruction throughout the body. This can lead to a protein-losing enteropathy, in particular.

More relevant to adult gastroenterologists is the secondary form of intestinal lymphangiectasia, in which some process affecting lymphatic outflow leads to diffuse lymphangiectasia of the small bowel mucosa. Heart failure is the most common reason for intestinal lymphangiectasia in adults. Other associations include abdominal malignancies, retroperitoneal fibrosis, abdominal tuberculosis, and sarcoidosis.

In this instance there is severe heart failure, leading to congestive hepatopathy (thus the elevated ALP, AST, and ALT), ascites, and intestinal lymphangiectasia. The white spots on endoscopy suggest dilated lacteals—a sign of underlying lymphangiectasia. The biopsies of lymphangiectasia reveal dilated lymphatics beneath the surface epithelium (see Figure 68-2). In addition, there may be a lymphocytic infiltration with villous injury—a pattern suggestive of celiac sprue. This injury can give rise to both protein and fat malabsorption. The decreased albumin is likely from protein malabsorption, and is very common in this condition. The low serum carotene and positive qualitative stool fat support fat malabsorption. The ascites may well be from heart failure, as suggested by the serum ascites albumin gradient (SAAG) >1.1.

Recall that a SAAG>1.1 suggests a transudative process like heart failure or cirrhosis, and a SAAG<1.1 suggests an exudative process like infection or malignancy. The total protein in heart failure is typically >2.5, whereas here it is lower (2.1). This might suggest cirrhosis, yet there are no stigmata of chronic liver disease on examination. Instead, the low ascitic protein is probably from protein-losing enteropathy resulting from the lymphangiectasia.

Why might this be tested? Malabsorption in general is common yet often poorly taught in GI training programs. We always think about celiac sprue as the most common form of malabsorption, and it is. But it is important to understand other causes of malabsorption. Although secondary intestinal lymphangiectasia is not common, it is not necessarily rare either. So examiners want to make sure you can identify the pathognomonic endoscopic findings, and can also keep it in mind when a patient with congestive heart failure (a common medical illness) presents with diarrhea (a common GI symptom).

Clinical Threshold Alert: If the SAAG is greater than 1.1, the ascites is likely from a transudative process (eg, cirrhosis, heart failure). If it is less than 1.1, it is likely from an exudative process (eg, infection, malignancy).

Figure 68-2.

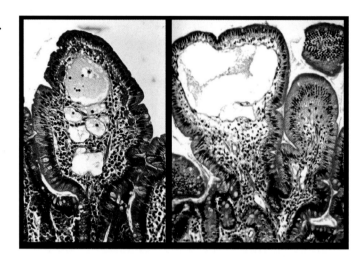

Here's the Point!

Low serum protein + Diarrhea + Focal white spots in small bowel = Intestinal Lymphangiectasia

Vignettes 69-79: Medication Adverse Event "Grab-Bag"

We use a lot of medications in GI and Hepatology. These can cause adverse events. In addition, common medications for non-GI conditions can affect the GI tract. For each "mini-vignette" below, identify the culprit medication and specify the related adverse event described in the scenario.

69. A patient with gastroparesis develops jaundice and pruritis shortly after beginning medical therapy for his recalcitrant nausea and vomiting.

70. The same patient, above, stops the first medication and starts another. She gets tongue-tied shortly after beginning the second therapy.

71. A patient develops painful swallowing while being treated for a chlamydial infection.

72. A nursing home patient with dementia is being treated for severe constipation. The patient aspirates while taking the medication, rapidly develops severe pneumonia, and dies.

73. A patient is using a short-course of high-dose therapy for an ankle sprain. He subsequently develops bloody diarrhea.

74. A patient receives a new medication for her seizure disorder. A month later she is found to have elevated liver tests. A subsequent liver biopsy reveals microvesicular steatosis.

75. A patient with longstanding RA develops hepatic fibrosis.

76. A young woman develops acute, sharp, right-upper quadrant pain. She is rushed to the Emergency Department where a CT scan reveals hemoperitoneum. Surgery fixes the problem. (This could be lots of things, but put on your "Board Hat," and think of a medication-induced complication that could explain this picture).

77. A patient with chronic migraine headache develops bloody diarrhea after taking a medication to halt a migraine attack.

78. A patient with cirrhosis is started on diuretic therapy for ascites. He subsequently develops severe abdominal pain, back pain, nausea, and vomiting.

79. Ridiculous "perfect storm" Board question: patient comes from Puerto Rico with diarrhea, malabsorption, and flat villi on biopsy—develops elevated liver enzymes after beginning therapy for his condition (name condition, medication, and side effect of medication).

Vignettes 69-79: Answers

69. This is erythromycin-induced cholestasis. Erythromycin is often used in gastroparesis to exploit its promotility benefits, rather than its antibiotic properties. Erythromycin is a motilin receptor agonist, which provides it some efficacy (albeit modest and often transient) in gastroparesis.

In any event, erythromycin can cause an acute cholestatic injury, typically seen biochemically with an ALP>2x the upper limit of normal, or an ALT/ALP ratio of <2. Drug induced cholestasis is traditionally divided into the "bland" type of pure canalicular injury, in which there is primarily an elevated ALP out of proportion to the liver enzymes, and so-called "hepatocanalicular" injury, in which the liver enzymes are also elevated along with the ALP.

The latter injury can be more serious than the pure canalicular pattern, since it often involves hepatocyte necrosis and destructive cholangitis. Unfortunately, erythromycin is more commonly associated with the hepatocanalicular pattern. Other drugs that cause hepatocanalicular injury include amoxicillin-clavulanate and chlorpromazine.

70. This is a metoclopramide-induced dystonic reaction. Although metoclopramide has reasonable efficacy in gastroparesis, it is highly limited by its prevalent and often severe neurological side effects. Extrapyramidal effects, such as tardive dyskinesia and dystonia, impact up to 30% of users. That is unbelievably common and should give you pause the next time you use metoclopramide. Still might be worth using (I sometimes use it), but always be wary of neurological side effects of this drug. In this case the "tongue tie" is a dystonic reaction.

71. This is doxycycline-induced esophagitis. Pill esophagitis can lead to severe odynophagia. The classic culprits include doxycycline, tetracycline, quinidine, aspirin, indomethacin, potassium, iron tablets, and alendronate. All of the medications must be taken with ample water, and should be consumed in the upright position. When these cause trouble, it is usually at areas of luminal narrowing, such as the crycopharyngeus (15 cm), compression of the aortic arch (20 to 23 cm), crossing of the left mainstem bronchus (25 to 27 cm), compression from the left atrium (26 to 28 cm), or at the lower esophageal sphincter (40 cm).

72. This is mineral oil-induced lipid pneumonia. Mineral oil is an emollient solution that can be very effective for constipation. However, it carries a grave risk for patients prone to aspirate. When inhaled, mineral oil can cause instant alveolar damage and result in lipid pneumonia. This can be fatal. So do not prescribe mineral oil to anyone who could possibly aspirate. It is not a good idea to use this in nursing home patients, for example.

73. This is NSAID-induced colitis. NSAIDs can cause an idiosyncratic colitis that mimics ischemic colitis. It presents clinically with lower abdominal pain and bloody diarrhea. As an aside, NSAIDs may also cause microscopic colitis (ie, collagenous colitis, lymphocytic colitis), although that relationship is not confirmed.

74. This is valproic acid induced microvesicular steatosis.

75. This is methotrexate (MTX)-induced hepatic fibrosis. Typically this would be identified well before fibrosis ensues, since patients on MTX require routine liver enzyme surveillance. If there is a spike in liver enzymes, then most providers would modify or discontinue MTX. In any event, MTX can cause hepatic fibrosis and even overt cirrhosis. As an aside, it is also associated with macrovesicular steatosis. What else causes macrovesicular steatosis, you ask? Here is another painful list to memorize: acetaminophen, cisplatin, corticosteroids, and tamoxifen.

76. This is estrogen-induced hepatic adenoma. As you probably remember from medical school, hepatic adenomas can be subcapsular, and can rupture and hemorrhage into the peritoneum. This can be a life-threatening event. This woman was probably taking oral contraceptives and subsequently developed an adenoma.

77. This is sumatriptan-induced ischemic colitis. Sumatriptan is one of several medications associated with ischemic colitis. Others include: alosetron, carboplatin, digitalis, diuretics, estrogens, NSAIDs, tegaserod, and paclitaxel. Cocaine is a "nonprescription" culprit.

78. This is furosemide-induced pancreatitis. There is a long list of medications associated with pancreatitis. Many are only loosely related, but some are more strongly linked. Here is a selected list of other strongly linked culprits: azathioprine, cimetidine, estrogens, 6-mercaptopurine, metronidazole, pentamidine, salicylates, sulfasalazine, sulfonamides, sulindac, tetracyclines, and valproic acid.

79. This is tetracycline-induced microvesicular steatosis. This patient has tropical sprue (see Vignette 66) and is being treated with tetracycline. Tetracycline, in turn, can lead to microvesicular steatosis. Other medications associated with microvesicular steatosis include aspirin (ie, Reye's syndrome), zidovudine (AZT), valproic acid, and vitamin A.

Why might this be tested? Because you just know it is going to be! This is one area you just have to learn—for tests and for life.

Medications that cause commonly-tested gastrointestinal and hepatic injuries are listed in Table 79-1. There are more drugs that could be included in each column, but these are the most common and/or most important examples.

Here's the Point!

| Learn Table 79-1! |

Table 79-1

MEDICATIONS THAT CAUSE GASTROINTESTINAL/HEPATIC INJURIES

Pill Esophagitis	Macrovesicular Steatosis	Microvesicular Steatosis	Ischemic Colitis	Pancreatitis
Alendronate	Acetaminophen	Aspirin	Alosetron	Azathioprine (AZA)
Aspirin	Cisplatin	Tetracycline	Carboplatin	Cimetidine
Doxycycline	Corticosteroids	Valproic acid	Cocaine	Estrogens
Indomethacin	Methotrexate	Vitamin A	Digitalis	Furosemide
Iron	Tamoxifen	Zidovudine (AZT)	Diuretics	6-mercaptopurine
Potassium			Estrogens	Metronidazole
Quinidine			NSAIDs	Pentamidine
			Tegaserod	Salicylates
			Paclitaxel	Sulfasalazine
				Sulindac
				Tetracycline
				Valproic Acid

Vignettes 80: Obstipation in the ICU

An 84-year-old woman with pneumonia on mechanical ventilation develops progressive abdominal distension and obstipation. An abdominal flat plate is obtained (Figure 80-1).

Figure 80-1. Abdominal flat plate for Vignette 74. (Used with permission from DiMarino AJ, Benjamin SB, eds. *Gastrointestinal Disease: An Endoscopic Approach.* Thorofare, NJ: SLACK Incorporated; 2002:901.)

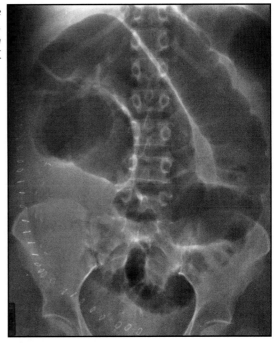

▸ **What is the most likely diagnosis?**

▸ **What is the first-line treatment?**

Vignette 80: Answer

This is acute colonic pseudo-obstruction, also known as Ogilvie's Syndrome. Ogilvie's syndrome is characterized by marked dilation of the cecum and ascending colon in the absence of mechanical obstruction (see Figure 80-1). Similar to ileus, colonic pseudo-obstruction generally occurs in critically ill patients with sepsis, recent surgery, electrolyte abnormalities, and trauma, among other conditions. The diagnosis rests on radiographic evaluation of the cecum, where a diameter of >10 to 12 cm predicts bowel perforation, and should serve as a critical threshold to track in patients with suspected pseudo-obstruction.

The clinical presentation of acute colonic pseudo-obstruction is typical of other obstructive processes, with the patient usually suffering marked abdominal distention, nausea, vomiting, and abdominal pain. If left untreated, colonic pseudo-obstruction can lead to ischemia, perforation (in approximately 3% of cases), peritonitis, and death. Thus, the clinician must keep a high index of suspicion for colonic pseudo-obstruction in patients with risk factors, as the consequences of late diagnosis can be grave.

Fortunately, conservative measures are sufficient in most cases of colonic pseudo-obstruction, and the cecal dilatation resolves spontaneously. Conservative measures consist of ceasing oral intake, frequent repositioning of the patient, and treating potential underlying causes of dysmotility (as with ileus). Although nasogastric tubes are often employed in colonic pseudo-obstruction, there are no data from randomized controlled studies to support its effectiveness in reducing clinically significant endpoints. In contrast, case series do support the effectiveness of colonoscopic decompression, which reduces the cecal diameter in upwards of 70% of patients. Unfortunately, colonic decompression alone is often short-lived, and recurrent distention occurs in nearly half of patients. Thus, colonic decompression is usually accompanied by placement of a rectal tube that is fed into the ascending colon (a maneuver that is easier said than done). Although colonoscopic decompression and rectal tube placement is conceptually attractive, it is practically a very difficult procedure to perform, since it must be conducted in an unprepared bowel (since bowel preparation is contraindicated in the setting of pseudo-obstruction) without the benefit of air insufflation (which could lead to perforation).

In patients failing to respond to conservative measures after 24 to 48 hours, including correction of electrolyte abnormalities, intravenous hydration, correction of underlying medical etiologies, and minimization of culprit medications, pharmacologic therapy is generally warranted. Moreover, if at any time the cecal diameter exceeds 12 cm, or if there is evidence of worsening clinical status, then aggressive treatment should be immediately pursued. Indeed, colonic pseudo-obstruction is a true GI emergency that warrants the involvement of a GI specialist regardless of the time of day. Given the shortcomings of colonic decompression, coupled with data that neostigmine appears highly effective in colonic pseudo-obstruction, the currently accepted first line therapy is intravenous neostigmine at a dosage of 2 mg intravenously times 1 infusion, followed by an additional 2 mg infusion 3 hours later if there is no initial response or adverse events. Because neostigmine is an anticholinesterase inhibitor, it is associated with typical cholinergic side effects, including bronchoconstriction, abdominal cramping, hypersalivation, diaphoresis, and bradycardia. Because cardiovascular collapse is possible (although generally transient and rarely life threatening), neostigmine must be administered in a monitored setting. It is contraindicated in patients with bradycardia, active bronchospasm, and mechanical bowel obstruction. In the rare situation of failure to respond to conservative measures, neostigmine, and colonic decompression, surgery is a last resort. However, surgery is highly morbid, and may lead to poor outcomes in patients who are already critically ill to begin with. Indeed, case series indicate that one-quarter of patients with colonic pseudo-obstruction die in the perioperative period, even in the absence of bowel perforation. Given these poor outcomes, it is unclear whether surgical treatment is warranted, especially since the risk of perforation in colonic pseudo-obstruction is thought to be around 3%.

Why might this be tested? Other than acute GI bleeding, there aren't too many true GI emergencies that demand attention at 3 AM. Foreign body ingestions, acute gallstone pancreatitis, and this—Ogilvie's Syndrome, round out most of the remaining 3 AM culprits that you can actually do something about (in contrast to caustic ingestions, acute post-polypectomy syndrome, etc—all bad, but not much you can do at 3 AM unfortunately). You should know about all of these treatable 3 AM emergencies.

Clinical Threshold Alert: If the cecal diameter exceeds 10 to 12 cm in Ogilvie's syndrome, then the risk of perforation increases significantly. Neostigmine is warranted in this setting.

Here's the Point!

ICU Patient with Obstipation and Dilated Cecum >10 cm = Ogilvie's Syndrome… think about neostigmine

Vignette 81: Chronic Cholecystitis and Small Bowel Obstruction

A 72-year-old woman with a history of chronic gallstone disease and recurrent cholecystitis presents to the emergency department with 4 hours of severe, unremitting abdominal pain. The pain is throughout her abdomen and comes in "waves." She has vomited several times. Examination reveals abdominal distension and high-pitched bowel sounds.

An abdominal radiograph reveals a 3-cm, irregular, opaque object in the sigmoid bowel with evidence of colonic obstruction (Figure 81-1). A follow-up abdominal CT scan confirms colonic obstruction and reveals an intraluminal object obstructing the sigmoid colon, along with evidence of pneumobilia and air within the gallbladder itself (Figure 81-1). Of note, there is no previous history of ERCP or sphincterotomy.

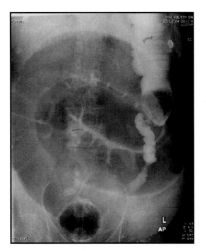 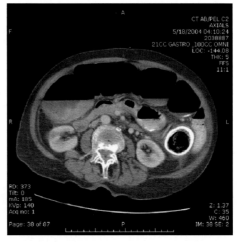

Figure 81-1. Abdominal imaging of patient in Vignette 81. (Used with permission from Jorge Obando, MD, Lahey Clinic, Burlington, MA.)

▶ *What is the most likely diagnosis?*

▶ *How did this happen?*

Vignette 81: Answer

This is gallstone ileus. Gallstone ileus results when a gallstone mechanically obstructs the intestines as a result of abnormal communication between the gallbladder and bowel. This usually occurs in the setting of chronic cholecystitis from gallstones. With chronic inflammation, gallstones can slowly erode through the wall of the gallbladder and directly into the intestines.

The most common communication is between the gallbladder and duodenum. When this happens, the stone usually gets caught at the ileocecal valve and leads to small bowel obstruction, assuming the stone is 2 cm or larger. Smaller stones are usually passed without significant obstruction.

This case has a twist, since there is a large stone in the sigmoid bowel that somehow bypassed the ileocecal valve. In this instance the stone eroded directly into the colon—not the duodenum. That is why there is a large bowel obstruction rather than the more common small bowel obstruction.

The presence of gallbladder air (called Balthazar's sign, by the way) indicates a direct communication between the gallbladder and intestines vs a gas-forming anaerobic infection like *Clostridium perfringens*. The latter seems unlikely given this presentation. There is no history of a sphincterotomy, which is the other risk factor for pneumobilia. Thus, the presence of air in the gallbladder and biliary tree, coupled with a large bowel obstruction from an opaque intraluminal mass, makes gallstone ileus the most likely explanation.

Treatment is surgical—both an enterotomy with stone retrieval and a cholecystectomy.

Why might this be tested? Board examiners have a bunch of content "check boxes" they need to click off when putting an exam together. This topic is convenient because it covers several areas, including biliary disorders, luminal pathology, and surgery. With one question they could potentially test across several content areas. Also, this condition sometimes goes undiagnosed for a while, particularly when patients have a "rolling obstruction" where the stone slowly passes downstream over several days. So it is important to make this diagnosis early and accurately, and examiners may want to confirm your ability to do so.

Clinical Threshold Alert: If a gallstone is larger than 2 cm, it will probably get stuck in the ileocecal valve and cause a small bowel obstruction. If it works its way into the colon, it may get stuck in the sigmoid colon (particularly if greater than 2.5 cm for colonic obstruction).

Here's the Point!

History of gallstones + Recurrent cholecystitis + Bowel obstruction + Air in Gallbladder = Gallstone Ileus

Vignettes 82-89: HIV and Diarrhea

The GI tract is one huge immune organ, so it is a major target for HIV. Diarrhea is one of the most common symptoms in HIV and AIDS, so it is important to be well versed in the differential diagnosis and treatment of HIV-related diarrhea. Below is a collection of "mini-vignettes" of patients with AIDS, CD4 counts below 200, and diarrhea. For each one, identify the culprit organism and specify the treatment.

82. Urgency, tenesmus, bloody diarrhea, and paresthesias in a "saddle" distribution.

83. CD4 of 50, with bloody diarrhea, high fevers, severe abdominal pain, and a CT scan revealing colitis and bulky intra-abdominal lymphadenopathy. Biopsies reveal "foamy macrophages" that are acid fast.

84. Bloody diarrhea with multiple "flask-shaped" colonic ulcers and motile trophozoites with ingested erythrocytes on wet mount of the stool.

85. Fever, weight loss, cough, diarrhea, and terminal ileitis.

86. Low-grade fever, voluminous watery diarrhea, cholecystitis, and terminal ileitis.

87. Bloody diarrhea and colonic ulcers with "owl's eye" inclusion bodies.

88. Voluminous diarrhea and eosinophilia after visiting a developing country.

89. Fever, watery diarrhea, low serum carotene, and enterocytes with PAS-positive acid-fast "foamy macrophages."

Vignettes 82-89: Answers

82. This is herpes simplex virus (HSV) proctitis. HSV is neurotropic, so it can lead to various forms of neuropathy. When it involves the sacral nerves (S2, S3, S4), it can lead to paresthesias in a "saddle" distribution. This is a rare but nearly pathognomonic feature of sacral HSV. The symptoms of urgency, tenesmus, and bloody stool output suggest proctitis. HSV does not typically cause a full colitis, but instead leads to a limited procto-sigmoiditis. Although not described here, patients may have perianal vesicles, along with ulcerative proctitis on sigmoidoscopy.

The differential diagnosis for proctitis, particularly in men who have sex with men, includes gonorrhea, HSV, chlamydia, mixed infections, and syphilis (*T. pallidum*), in order of decreasing prevalence. Treatment is with anti-HSV treatments, such as acyclovir, famciclovir, or valacyclovir.

83. This is MAC colitis. MAC is the most common systemic bacterial infection in HIV patients. It is most common with the CD4≤50. MAC can involve nearly every organ system, so it is another one of these diagnoses that you can offer in the differential diagnosis of just about anything and probably be in the ballpark. When it involves the GI tract, its most common manifestation is colitis, which can be severe or even fulminant.

The other 2 organisms that can lead to fulminant colitis in AIDS include CMV and *E. histolytica*. Clinically, MAC-related colitis presents with severe abdominal pain, high fevers, night sweats, and bloody diarrhea. The ulcers in MAC can become deep and even perforate in severe cases. There is often bulky intra-abdominal lymphadenopathy, which can also contribute to the abdominal pain. On histology, there are "foamy macrophages" stuffed with the organism that are acid fast. Treatment is with anti-TB agents, like ethambutol or rifabutin, typically in combination with clarithromycin or azithromycin.

84. This is *Entamoeba histolytica* colitis. Amoebic colitis can be severe in HIV. *E. histolytica* is one of the "big three" organisms that can lead to fulminant colitis, along with MAC and CMV. *E. histolytica* can present across a wide clinical range, including noninvasive asymptomatic colonization, self-limited diarrhea, colitis, and fulminant colitis. The latter can lead to toxic megacolon and perforation, which is usually heralded by bloody diarrhea with worsening abdominal pain. Over time, chronic colitis can lead to stricture formation. The organisms may invade the mucosa and work their way into the portal circulation, enter the liver, and lead to the formation of amoebic liver abscesses.

The diagnosis requires a wet mount of stool specimens, which reveal motile trophozoites with characteristic ingested erythrocytes. Colonoscopy may reveal nonspecific colitis with characteristic flask-shaped ulcers in the mucosa—a fanciful descriptor indicating that the ulcers have a narrow neck and a wide base, like a pouring flask. When the symptoms are severe, colonoscopy is relatively contraindicated given the risk of perforation in fulminant *E. histolytica* colitis. Treatment is with metronidazole followed by paramomycin or iodoquinol.

85. This is gastrointestinal tuberculosis (TB). Like MAC, tuberculosis can affect virtually every organ system, including the GI tract. For whatever reason,

TB often affects the terminal ileum, which is a tip-off in this vignette. Of note, cryptosporium can also colonize the terminal ileum, but the picture in this vignette is not otherwise suggestive of crypto. Intestinal TB can mimic Crohn's Disease—ie, abdominal pain, weight loss, and ulcerated terminal ileitis. In this case the history of HIV positivity, coupled with the cough, suggests TB rather than Crohn's Disease. Colonoscopy can reveal a wide range of lesions, including ulcers, strictures, fistulae, nodules, and a deformed ileocecal valve. Treatment is with typical anti-TB drugs, and is similar to the treatment of pulmonary TB. Treatment is usually effective. Surgery is reserved for patients with structural complications (strictures, fistulae) or rare perforations.

86. This is cryptosporidiosis. Refer to Vignette 7 for further information.

87. This is CMV colitis. CMV is one of the "big three" that can lead to severe, fulminant colitis with toxic megacolon (others: *E. histolytica* and MAC). Of course, CMV can affect the entire GI tract, along with nearly every other organ system. CMV is most common when the CD4≤100. In addition to colitis, CMV can lead to enteritis and present with voluminous nonbloody diarrhea.

The characteristic pathophysiology involves vasculitis and thrombosis of intraluminal arterioles with occlusion and ischemia (it is no wonder this can be such a fulminant disease). The diagnosis rests upon endoscopic biopsy; stool studies are not available and serology and viral loads are not highly sensitive or specific (most HIV patients already have positive titers). The colonoscopic appearance of CMV is variable—it can really look like anything. There may be diffuse erythema and friability with characteristically discrete ulcers with clean bases. The ulcers may also be serpiginous. The ulcers can occur anywhere in the colon, but are commonly in the right colon. Therefore, a flexsig is not adequate to assess for CMV colitis.

In general, you should take 4 quadrant biopsies every 10 cm across all segments of the colon, since the CMV organisms may be found in both abnormal and normal tissue—so be liberal, because you never know exactly where you'll find it. When sampling an ulcer, be sure to take the biopsy from the center—not just the rim. Because CMV tends to invade the blood vessels, and since the vessels tend to reside at the deepest part of the ulcers, a central biopsy can maximize the yield for CMV. This is in contrast to HSV, which tends to live on the rim of the ulcer (surface dwellers). These biopsy principles also pertain to esophageal ulcers, by the way, where CMV and HSV are the usually 2 top suspects when faced with esophageal ulcers. Again, biopsy in the **C**enter for **C**MV, and **H**igh on the rim for **H**SV (see Vignette 147 for more on this). Histology typically reveals the characteristic "owls' eye" appearance corresponding with intranuclear inclusion bodies.

Treatment is with 3 to 5 weeks of intravenous gancyclovir, foscarnet, or a combination of both. Be sure to also check the eyes in anyone with systemic CMV—people forget to do that.

88. This is isospora belli enteritis. It is hard to keep track of all the GI parasites in AIDS. The usual suspects include cryptosporidium, microspora, isospora, and cyclospora. Of these, cryptosporidium is the most prevalent and, thus, the most important (both for Boards and for life). But isospora tends to show up every now and then (also for Boards and for life). The tip-off here is the recent travel to a developing country (typically Africa or Haiti), coupled with the eosinophilia. It is extremely rare in the United States. The typical clinical picture is like crypto, only milder. There can be Charcot-Leyden crystals in the stool (Board buzzword). As with crypto, diagnosis of isospora relies on acid fast staining of the stools to detect oocysts, which are generally much larger than those of crypto. On endoscopic biopsy the organisms can be found in the brush border, as with crypto, but also within intracytoplasmic vacuoles, unlike with crypto. Finally, unlike crypto, isospora is exquisitely sensitive to trimethoprim-sulfamethoxazole (TMP-SMX). In fact, the high rates of TMP-SMX prophylaxis for *pneumocystis carinii* in the United States may explain the low incidence of isospora compared with other countries.

89. This is MAC enteritis. The low serum carotene and watery diarrhea suggests diffuse small bowel malabsorption. MAC can stuff itself into macrophages in the foregut enterocytes, leading to PAS-positive, acid-fast, "foamy macrophages." Of note, Whipple's Disease, a perennial Board review favorite, can also present with diarrhea, malabsorption, and PAS-positive foamy macrophages stuffed full of the *Tropheryma whippelii* organism. However, the foamy macrophages of Whipple's disease are not acid-fast. Of course, in a patient with AIDS, Whipple's does not come straight to the top of the differential diagnosis anyway.

Here's the Point!

HIV, Diarrhea and...
Foamy macrophages = MAC (unlikely Whipple's)
Flask-shaped ulcers = *E. histolytica*
Charcot-Leyden crystals = *Isospora*
Owl's Eyes = CMV
Saddle Paresthesia = HSV
Terminal Ileitis = Crypto or TB
Trophozoites with ingested RBCs = *E. histolytica*
Fulminant Colitis = CMV, *E. histolytica*, MAC
Africa or Haiti = *Isospora*

Vignette 90: Acute Abdominal Pain with Something on CT

A 24-year-old woman presents to the emergency department with acute-onset abdominal pain. She was in her usual state of excellent health until, while sitting and watching television, she experienced an abrupt onset of dull, "achy" pain in her left lower quadrant. The pain began 8 hours prior to arrival, and has been persistent ever since. The pain does not radiate. It does not change with positioning.

There is no diarrhea, bloody BMs, nausea, vomiting, vaginal discharge, dysuria, cloudy urine, fever, chills, sweats, or other systemic symptoms. She does not take aspirin, NSAIDs, or any other medications. Her last menstrual period was 1 week ago. She has no history of a similar pain.

On examination her vital signs are unremarkable; there is no fever. She is tender to light palpation in the left lower quadrant, and demonstrates voluntary guarding. There is no rebound, involuntary guarding, or other peritoneal signs. Pelvic examination reveals a normal appearing cervix without motion tenderness. There is no cervical discharge. Her leukocyte count is slightly elevated at 13, with 75% neutrophils. She is not anemic, has a normal platelet count, normal electrolytes, and a normal BUN and creatinine. Urinalysis is normal.

A CT scan is performed, which reveals a normal cecum and appendix, and no diverticula. In the anti-mesenteric border of the sigmoid colon there is a focal oval area of fat with inflammatory stranding and a linear, central attenuating line through the inflamed fat.

▶ **What is the diagnosis?**

▶ **Does this need surgery?**

Vignettes 90: Answer

This is epiploic appendagitis. You might remember learning about the epiploic appendages back in medical school. These are the little fat tags that line the anti-mesenteric border of the colon. Although they are present along the entire length of the colon, they are usually more dense, larger, and longer in the transverse and sigmoid colon. Because these project into the peritoneal cavity, they can easily cause abdominal pain if they become inflamed or necrosed.

That is exactly what happened in this vignette. These appendages can twist and turn, particularly when abnormally elongated, which can lead to torsion of the penetrating vessels and lymphatics. This acute strangulation produces transient ischemia or even infarction of the fat tag, which causes acute and localized abdominal pain.

The presentation is similar to a wide range of other intra-abdominal processes, and is frequently mistaken for acute appendicitis, particularly when involving the ascending colon. Rebound tenderness and peritoneal signs are rare because the affected tissue is so small and localized. Other systemic symptoms, like fevers or sweats, are also rare. There may be a mildly elevated white count, as seen in this vignette, but not much more than that. The pain is more commonly in the left than the right lower quadrant, since the longer appendages (ie, more likely to torse) are in the sigmoid bowel.

The CT scan may reveal the pathognomonic findings seen in this vignette—namely, focal oval area of fat with inflammatory stranding and a linear, central attenuating line through the inflamed fat. The central line, when present, corresponds with a thrombosed penetrating vein. Abdominal ultrasound may also find the lesion.

Treatment is conservative—not surgery. Some use high dose anti-inflammatory drugs like NSAIDs. But most patients can go home, take oral medications, and totally avoid surgery. Because this is a self-limiting process, it is important to avoid performing surgery, which may well be an option on an exam.

Why might this be tested? Because it is rare, but actually does happen. The main point is to be able to recognize the pathognomonic radiographic findings, understand that the natural history is benign, and avoid surgery. Board examiners want to make sure you don't let people die (subject of other questions), but also don't want you to perform unnecessary and potentially harmful maneuvers (eg, surgery) if not warranted. This question falls in the latter group.

Here's the Point!

Acute Abdominal Pain (especially left-sided) + Focal Oval Area of Fat on CT = Epiploic Appendagitis

Vignette 91: More Abdominal Pain

A 42-year-old man presents with chronic abdominal pain. The pain began 12 years ago, and first developed after undergoing a ventral hernia repair. He explains that the pain is near his surgical site, and points to the right of his umbilicus. He describes the pain as sharp, worse with sitting up, and present nearly every day. The pain is unrelated to meals. There is no nausea, vomiting, early satiety or bloating. There is no diarrhea, constipation, or bloody BMs. He does not take aspirin or NSAIDs.

He has undergone a barrage of diagnostic tests over the years, including upper endoscopy, colonoscopy, capsule endoscopy, CT scanning, and abdominal ultrasonography. These tests have been unrevealing. The symptoms did not improve with a trial of PPI therapy. He was diagnosed with IBS and placed on a tricyclic antidepressant medication, which has not improved the pain.

On examination his vital signs are normal. He has sharp tenderness along the right side of his rectus sheath, near his surgical scar. The pain is discrete and localized. The patient is asked to perform a half sit-up during palpation of the tender site, and this worsens the pain markedly. The remainder of his examination is unremarkable, and all of his laboratory values are normal.

▸ **What is the diagnosis?**

▸ **What is the treatment?**

Vignette 91: Answer

This is abdominal wall pain, likely from anterior cutaneous nerve entrapment syndrome. The pathophysiology of this condition remains somewhat of a mystery, but the idea is that the anterior cutaneous nerves from T7-T11 may become entrapped as they enter the fibrous ring along the lateral border of the rectus sheath. Scar tissue, in particular, may cause entrapment—a consequence of previous abdominal surgery. Abdominal wall pain is often (but not always) right sided, within a few centimeters of the rectus abdominis muscle, and highly localized—typically 1 or 2 fingertips in area.

The Carnett maneuver can help distinguish between abdominal wall and visceral pain. The idea is simple. Both abdominal wall and visceral pain get worse with palpation. So, the first thing you need to do is locate the point of maximal tenderness. Then, while exerting pressure on the tender point, ask the patient to perform a half sit-up by contracting the abdominal musculature. If this makes the pain worse, then the test is positive for abdominal wall pain. If the pain improves, then it suggests a visceral source. The concept is that visceral pain will be alleviated with abdominal wall contraction, since the contracted muscles form a barrier between the examiner's hand and the underlying diseased viscera. So the barrier reduces the downward pressure on the viscera, and the pain improves.

In contrast, when the pain arises from the abdominal wall itself, the pain becomes worse with contraction—not better, as occurs with visceral pain. In this case the patient has a positive Carnett maneuver. Together with the classic history and proximity of the pain to the abdominal scar, the diagnosis is almost certainly abdominal wall pain. This is often misdiagnosed, and patients can go years without the proper treatment, which is abdominal wall injection.

The typical therapy is to inject 3 mL of a 1% lidocaine or xylocaine solution into the point of maximal tenderness, typically at a right angle to the abdominal wall and deep enough to get into the muscle layer. If this provides a benefit, then it should be followed up with 20 to 40 mg of a long-acting steroid like triamcinolone.

When this works, it really works—usually within minutes. We do this quite often in our teaching clinic at UCLA, and I can attest that it really works. We have had patients with years of pain practically dance a jig after getting the injection. We are still waiting for a proper randomized controlled trial vs something like a saline sham—but until then, we inject. And that is what you should do on a Board question as well.

Why might this be tested? Because patients can go for years misdiagnosed and mistreated. It is up to you to think about this condition, both on Boards and in real life, and to know about the Carnett maneuver. And there is nothing more satisfying that curing years of abdominal pain with a simple abdominal injection. Many clinicians don't know about this, so that is why it is perfect fodder for the Board exam.

Here's the Point!

Acute abdominal pain (especially right sided and focal) + Positive Carnett Maneuver = Abdominal Wall Pain

Vignette 92: Severe Abdominal Pain After Exercise

An 18-year-old college student of Armenian descent presents to the emergency department of his University's Medical Center with acute, severe, diffuse abdominal pain. He was in his usual state of health until 3 hours before presentation, when he developed a paroxysmal attack of abdominal pain, described as "all over" and "nonstop." It does not radiate beyond the abdomen.

Earlier in the day he participated in a cross-country race as a member of the University team. He now complains of feeling sweaty, feverish, and nauseous. He has not vomited. There has been no diarrhea or bloody stools. He does not take aspirin, NSAIDs, or other medications. He denies use of illicit drugs. There have been no previous episodes like this one. However, he recalls having acute, severe chest pain 1 year ago for which he sought care, but never received a clear diagnosis. The episode was transient and has not returned. He reports a family history of "abdominal problems," but does not know more than that.

On exam he appears in extremis, and is writhing in pain in bed. Vital signs: temperature=100.8; heart rate=110; respiratory rate=16; blood pressure=138/90. His abdominal exam reveals a diffusely tender abdomen, involuntary guarding, and rebound tenderness. Rectal examination is unremarkable. There is a patch of tender, erythematous skin along his right ankle and the dorsum of his right foot. The remainder of his examination is unrevealing. Abnormal labs include an elevated white count of 14.8 (92% PMNs) and an ESR of 68. A CT scan of the abdomen does not identify a culprit organ or other focal abnormality.

▶ **What is the diagnosis?**

▶ **Is his ethnicity relevant?**

▶ **Is it time for exploratory laparotomy?**

Vignette 92: Answer

This is an acute attack of Familial Mediterranean Fever, or FMF. FMF is an unusual, pro-inflammatory condition that is most common in ethnic groups from the Mediterranean, including Armenians, Sephardic Jews, North Africans, Arabs, Turks, Greeks, and Italians. FMF is an autosomal recessive disorder with incomplete penetrance.

The culprit gene is called, aptly enough, the FMF gene, and is found on chromosome 16. The gene encodes a protein called pyrin, which is a transcription regulator for pro-inflammatory peptides like interleukin-1 beta, among others. When pyrin is dysregulated, a pro-inflammatory state can develop, leading to a range of clinical symptoms including peritonitis, pleuritis, arthritis, and cellulitis-like skin lesion (that is not, in fact, cellulitis—but that mimics cellulitis). Most patients have their first attack before the age of 20, as occurred here. Nobody knows what can trigger an attack, but stress and exercise have been implicated. In this case the patient developed his bout after running a cross country race.

The clinical picture can be indistinguishable from an acute abdomen, and many patients proceed to exploratory laparotomy to search for the usual suspects, like appendicitis, cholecystitis, etc. The presentation can be very dramatic, and wholly compatible with acute appendicitis or other severe intra-abdominal processes.

In this case, however, the ethnic background, family history of "abdominal problems," paroxysmal onset after exercise, history of a pleuritis-like episode, presence of a cellulitis-like lesion on the right ankle, and elevated ESR all point towards FMF. Although it might be hard to resist the urge to bring this patient to the operating room, it would ultimately yield nothing.

The best treatment is to begin colchicine, which is the only consistently effective treatment for acute FMF. Of note, longstanding FMF can lead to secondary amyloidosis, which itself can be devastating (see Vignette 2 for more on amyloid). Colchicine prophylaxis may reduce not only the frequency of subsequent attacks, but also renal failure and other consequences of unchecked amyloidosis.

Here's the Point!

Young patient of Mediterranean origin with intermittent bouts of overwhelming abdominal pain, elevated ESR, and family history of the same = FMF

Vignette 93: Long-Term Constipation in a Young Man

A 20-year-old man is referred to you for longstanding, severe constipation. He has suffered from constipation for as long as he can remember. His primary symptoms include excessive straining, infrequent bowel movements (less than 3 per week on average), and occasional need for rectal digital manipulation to help in evacuation of stool. He has taken a range of laxatives, including stool softeners, fiber, and senna—all without success. A recent colonoscopy revealed only internal hemorrhoids and evidence of melanosis coli. His CBC, electrolytes, glucose, and TSH are all normal. He is not receiving any medications that could promote constipation. You decide to perform anorectal manometry with balloon inflation. Figure 93-1 is the manometric tracing that results after the rectal balloon is inflated with 60 cc of saline—the patient is not attempting to expel the balloon at this time.

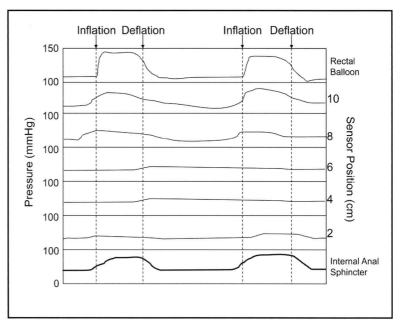

Figure 93-1. Anorectal manometry tracing during balloon inflation-deflation cycles.

▶ **What is the diagnosis?**

▶ **What is the definitive treatment?**

Vignette 93 Answer

This is adult Hirschprung's Disease. Hirschprung's Disease arises from failure of the neural crest cells to migrate to the end of the bowel during normal embryogenesis. This results in an aganglionic segment of bowel that is dysfunctional. The disease is characterized by a lack of reflex inhibition of the internal anal sphincter due to lack of enteric inhibitory neurons. The segment may be long, in which case the disease is typically detected shortly after birth in neonates who are unable to pass meconium. But short segments of Hirschprung's Disease may evade detection for years, and only present with longstanding constipation.

In this case, the patient had constipation for as long as he can remember, suggesting that this is not a run of the mill situation and there may be something organic. Of course, there are many conditions that can cause longstanding constipation, but when the symptoms fail to respond to a series of medical maneuvers, it's worth thinking a little harder about what might be underlying the problem. Anorectal manometry can be useful to rule out the rare but important conditions like adult Hirshprung's Disease or the much more common (yet still somewhat rare) pelvic dyssynergia (see Vignette 24 for details).

It might be easy to confuse this picture for pelvic dyssynergia. In Hirshprung's Disease, there is a lack of relaxation of the internal anal sphincter upon rectal balloon inflation to 40 to 60 cc. The normal, evolutionarily-sound reflex is for the internal anal sphincter to relax when a bowel movement enters the rectal vault. This is under autonomic control, in contrast to the external anal sphincter which is under voluntary control. The external anal sphincter normally remains closed when a stool enters the rectal vault, allowing us to pick and choose when and where to defecate (thankfully). So in Hirshprung's, the internal anal sphincter fails to automatically relax upon distension of the proximal rectum, as emulated by the balloon inflation in Figure 93-1. In pelvic dyssynergia, the problem is paradoxical contraction of the external anal sphincter upon attempted balloon expulsion. That is depicted in Figure 24-1 earlier in the book. But in this case, the patient is not even yet attempting to defecate. Instead, the internal (not external) anal sphincter is contracting when it should should be relaxing.

The diagnosis of Hirschprung's can be confirmed with a full thickness rectal biopsy. The classic finding is a lack of neurons (aganglionosis) in the affected segment. When this is confirmed, the next step, assuming there is truly a functional deficit, is to refer the patient for surgery. The goal is to remove the aganglionic segments and to then bring down normal tissue to restore continuity with the anus.

Here's the Point!

Longstanding constipation with no internal anal sphincter relaxation during rectal balloon inflation = Hirschprung's Disease

Vignettes 94-101: Subepithelial Gastric Mass Round-Up

Subepithelial masses are commonly found during upper endoscopy. The differential diagnosis for these lesions is lengthy. We usually establish the diagnosis using a combination of size, endoscopic appearance, EUS echotexture and location, and, in some cases, biopsy with immunostaining. For each mini-vignette, below, provide the likely lesion and the treatment plan.

94. A 3.5-cm subepithelial mass is found in the stomach during upper endoscopy for dyspepsia. EUS reveals a hypoechoic 4th layer tumor. Biopsy with immunostaining reveals c-kit (CD 117) positivity.

95. A 1-cm subepithelial mass is found in the stomach during upper endoscopy for dyspepsia. EUS reveals a hypoechoic 4th layer tumor. Biopsy with immunostaining reveals actin positivity, but negative c-kit staining.

96. A 2-cm subepithelial mass is found in the stomach during upper endoscopy for evaluation of iron deficiency anemia. The endoscopy is otherwise normal. Subsequent EUS reveals an extramural, anechoic, spherical structure at the site of the subepithelial bulge.

97. A 2-cm subepithelial mass is found in the stomach during upper endoscopy for reflux symptoms. The mass demonstrates a "pillow sign," meaning that it indents with pressure from the forceps, and slowly reforms upon withdrawal of the forceps. Subsequent EUS reveals a hyperechoic, well circumscribed, 3rd layer tumor.

98. Several subepithelial masses are found in the stomach during upper endoscopy for dyspepsia in the setting of a previous Billroth II procedure for peptic ulcer disease. The gastrin is also elevated, and a secretin stimulation test is negative. The subepithelial masses range in size from a subcentimeter to 2 cm, and are scattered throughout the stomach. Subsequent EUS reveals the lesions to be in the 2nd and 3rd layers of the stomach wall and hypoechoic in echotexture.

99. A 1.5-cm subepithelial mass is found in the stomach during upper endoscopy for dyspepsia. EUS reveals a hypoechoic 4th layer tumor. Biopsy with immunostaining reveals actin and vimentin positivity, but c-kit negativity.

100. A 2-cm subepithelial mass is found in the stomach during upper endoscopy for dyspepsia. EUS reveals a hypoechoic 4th layer tumor. Biopsy with immunostaining reveals S-100 positivity.

101. A 2-cm subepithelial prepyloric mass is found in the antrum of the stomach during upper endoscopy for dyspepsia. The mass has a central umbilication. EUS reveals a hypoechoic mass arising from the third sonographic layer (Figure 94-1).

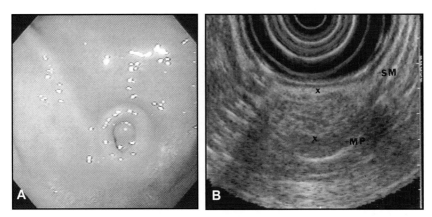

Figure 94-1. A) reveals a lesion in the antrum with a central umbilication. B) displays the lesion when viewed with EUS. (Used with permission from Firas H. Al-Kawas, MD, Georgetown University Hospital, Washington, DC.)

Vignettes 94-101: Answers

Before we work through the answers, it is first important to review the endoscopic layers of the stomach. There are usually 5 layers seen on EUS, as described in Figure 94-2.

The first and second layers jointly comprise the epithelium. Specifically, the first layer, which appears white, or "hyperechoic," is produced from signal coupling between the mucosal surface and the ultrasound waves. It is called the superficial epithelial layer. The second layer, which probably corresponds with the muscularis mucosae (not the muscularis propria, which comes later), is the deep epithelial layer. It appears dark, or "hypoechoic," on EUS. The muscularis mucosae is the usual dividing layer for an ulcer. That is, "ulcers" that do not penetrate the muscularis mucosae are considered erosions, not ulcers. A lesion becomes an ulcer once it penetrates the muscularis mucosae.

In any event, the third endoscopic layer corresponds with the submucosa, and is light. It correlates with the lamina propria. The fourth endoscopic layer is thick and dark, and corresponds with the muscularis propria. This is the most common layer in which subepithelial gastric masses arise.

Finally, the fifth layer is the serosa. It appears light. So there is a "light-dark-light-dark-light" pattern. Just remember that it starts with the "light" and ends with "light" ("...let there be light"). Figure 94-2 provides a typical EUS cross-section of the gastric layers. Be sure you are familiar with this. It is unlikely that you will be asked complex or nuanced questions about EUS imaging, but knowing the layers and identifying which layer harbors a tumor is certainly fair game.

Figure 94-2. Endoscopic ultrasound layers of the stomach and their correlation with the histological layer. There are alternating hyperechoic (white) and hypoechoic (dark) bands. (Used with permission from DiMarino AJ, Benjamin SB, eds. *Gastrointestinal Disease: An Endoscopic Approach.* Thorofare, NJ: SLACK Incorporated; 2002:384.)

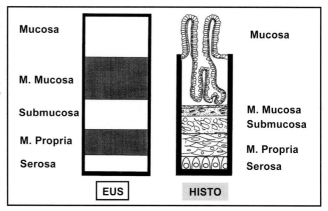

94. This is a gastrointestinal stromal tumor, or GIST. GISTs are the most common intramural lesion of the stomach. We used to think these were simple leiomyomas, but it turns out GISTs are different. Whereas leiomyomas arise from smooth muscle cells and stain positive for smooth muscle actin on immunohistochemistry, GISTs arise from the interstitial cells of Cajal (go figure), and stain positive for CD117, also known as c-kit—a tyrosine kinase receptor that is the target of imatinib mesylate (aka Gleevac, Novartis, East Hanover, NJ).

These tumors tend to occur in the mid-stomach and are usually smooth on endoscopic appearance. On occasion they may break through the mucosa and ulcerate—a potentially ominous sign, although not necessarily indicative of malignancy. On EUS they most often arise from the 4th layer, and less frequently arise from the 2nd layer. This makes sense, since both the 2nd and 4th layers are muscular, and GISTs arise from muscle layers. Since they arise from the 2nd and 4th layers, they are hypoechoic by EUS echotexture.

It is important to keep in mind that 10% to 30% of these lesions may harbor underlying malignancy, so they are not benign lesions like leiomyomas. Signs of malignancy include heterogenous echotexture, irregular margins, cystic spaces, size exceeding 4 cm, and perigastric lymph nodes exceeding 1 cm.

In contrast, benign lesions tend to have homogenous echotexture, smooth margins, no associated lymph nodes, and are smaller than 3 cm. Of note, there are definitely reports of underlying malignancy even in GISTs that are small, smooth, and well-demarcated. This is concerning, and has led to a debate about whether or not to surgically resect all GIST lesions. But setting the debate aside, you should plan to remove any lesion exceeding 3 cm in diameter, and any lesion that manifests other features concerning for malignancy (unless the tumor is already metastatic). So this lesion should be resected. Metastatic lesions may benefit from imatinib mesylate.

Here's the Point!

CD117 Positive + 4th Layer Subepithelial Mass = GIST

95. This is a gastric leiomyoma. This lesion can be endoscopically and ultrasonographically indistinguishable from a GIST tumor. But the difference, as noted above, is the result of immunostaining. Whereas GISTs stain positive for CD117, leiomyomas stain negative for CD117 but stain positive for smooth muscle actin. This is a small lesion that should not be removed—it should be monitored with EUS surveillance (exact surveillance intervals not evidence-based).

Here's the Point!

Actin Positive + CD117 Negative + 4th Layer Subepithelial Mass = Leiomyoma

96. This is a duplication cyst. Duplication cysts are rare embryological remnants from an accessory stomach. They are characteristically extramural, indicating that they arise from outside of the primary stomach. They are ultrasonographically spherical and anechoic. When large, these can lead to obstructions, although that is more common with small intestinal duplication cysts, since the lumen in the small bowel is much narrower than the stomach. These cysts can grow carcinoids and even gastric cancer—although the risk is not thought to be higher than the primary stomach. If there are obstructive symptoms, then the cyst should either be surgically removed (if large), or endoscopically drained (if smaller and near the gastric wall).

Here's the Point!

Spherical + Anechoic + Subepithelial Gastric Mass = Duplication Cyst

97. This is a lipoma. Lipomas are common, so you have probably seen these before. They are usually yellowish, and easily indent with pressure from a biopsy forcep. The "pillow sign" means that the indentation stays for a moment after removing the probe, and then slowly reforms and fills it. It is sort of like a pillow—when you have been lying on a pillow all night, the impression of your head remains even after you get up. It fills in thereafter. Lipomas are hyperechoic, well circumscribed, and typically arise from the 3rd layer. They are benign and no treatment is necessary.

Here's the Point!

Yellowish Mass + Pillow Sign = Lipoma

98. These are carcinoid tumors. Carcinoids arise from enterochromaffin-like (ECL) cells, and can be found throughout the GI tract. They usually arise from the mucosal layer and invade deeper planes as they grow. On EUS they are hypoechoic and are in the second or third layers. They can be multiple, as occurred here, or solitary. They are more commonly multiple in the setting of hypergastrinemia, since gastrin stimulates growth of carcinoid tumors.

In this vignette there is measurable hypergastrinemia and a negative secretin stimulation test, suggesting that the diagnosis is not ZES. The history of a Billroth II procedure suggests possible retained antrum syndrome. See Vignettes 29-33 for more about hypergastrinemia

In any event, carcinoids are classified as Types 1 through 3, where Type 1 (most common) is associated with hypergastrinemia from chronic atrophic gastritis. Type 2 occurs with ZES. Type 3 is sporadic and occurs with normal gastrin levels. Types 1 and 2 are considerably more benign than Type 3 lesions. The 5-year survival with Type 1 carcinoids is more than 95%, whereas up to 50% of Type 3 lesions can become malignant and metastasize. Because even small Type 3 carcinoids can become malignant, guidelines suggest removing these surgically even when small. For Type 1 and 2 carcinoids, most recommend endoscopic resection of small lesions (eg, 1 to 2 cm) followed by endoscopic surveillance.

Here's the Point!

Gastric Mass + 2nd or 3rd Layer + ECL Cells = Carcinoid

99. This is a glomus tumor. These tumors arise from smooth muscle cells from blood vessels. Although they typically occur outside of the GI tract, they can rarely present as subepithelial gastric masses when arising from the gastric wall. On EUS they appear hypoechoic and arise from the 4th layer (muscularis propria). This is similar to GIST tumors and leiomyomas, so you need more information to tell them apart.

Once again, the immunostaining can help you distinguish. In this case, the staining is positive for smooth muscle actin, as with leiomyomas, but also for vimentin. They are c-kit (CD-117) negative, distinguishing them from GISTs. Glomus tumors are almost always benign, but can rarely undergo malignant transformation. There are no explicit guidelines on how to manage this lesion. Given its size, endoscopic resection with subsequent surveillance is reasonable. But since the evidence is lacking, it would seem unlikely to get a question on how to manage a gastric glomus tumor (as opposed to making the diagnosis in the first place, which is certainly fair game).

Here's the Point!

Gastric Mass + 4th Layer + Vimenten Positive = Glomus Tumor

100. This is a schwannoma. Schwannomas arise form neural tissue, and are hypoechoic on EUS. They typically arise from the 4th layer, and stain positive for S-100 on immunohistochemistry.

Here's the Point!

Gastric Mass + 4th Layer + S-100 Positive = Schwannoma

101. This is most likely a pancreatic rest, or ectopic pancreatic tissue in the stomach. Pancreatic rests are most commonly found in the prepyloric antrum, and usually have a characteristic central umbilication. They are benign and do not require resection.

Here's the Point!

Prepyloric Mass + Central Umblication = Pancreatic Rest

Vignettes 102-109: Dysphagia Run-Down

Below is a collection of "mini-vignettes" describing patients with varying types of esophageal dysfunction. For each vignette, name the likely condition, and describe what manometric features would be found if each underwent traditional esophageal manometry.

102. A 17-year-old girl, who is a recent immigrant from Mexico, presents with dysphagia for solids and liquids. The symptoms began 3 months ago. She recalls swelling around her left eye prior to the onset of symptoms. She had been living in a thatched roof hut in Mexico.

103. A 72-year-old man presents with recent onset dysphagia for solids and liquids. This came "nearly overnight." He also has new-onset constipation. He has never before suffered either dysphagia or constipation. He has a 50-pack-year smoking history, and recently noticed an increasingly hoarse voice.

104. A 40-year-old woman complains of paroxysmal bouts of severe chest pain. She is unable to swallow any liquid or solid during these attacks. Between attacks she is fine, and does not suffer from dysphagia. Her cardiac evaluation has been totally normal.

105. A 50-year-old woman presents with progressive dysphagia for solids and liquids. She has difficulty standing from a seated position, and describes a violaceous rash, like a "shawl," at the nape of her neck.

106. A 50-year-old man presents with progressive weakness and atrophy of his lower extremity musculature, along with progressive dysphagia for solids and liquids. He had childhood polio at the age of 15.

107. A 32-year-old woman presents with progressive dysphagia, first for solids, then for solids and liquids. She has a "megaduodenum" on small bowel follow-through, and has recurrent bouts of small intestinal bacterial overgrowth.

108. An 83-year-old man presents with long-standing dysphagia. He explains that solid food is intermittently stuck in the "back of his throat," just as he is trying to swallow. There is no dysphagia to liquids. He has a history of osteoarthritis, along with repetitive traumatic neck injuries.

109. A 72-year-old woman presents with long-standing dysphagia to solids, but not liquids. The dysphagia has not been progressive. She remembers symptoms going back for at least a decade. She has no unintentional weight loss, no vomiting, no early satiety, and no significant constitutional symptoms. She has no oropharyngeal symptoms of note. Her primary care physician ordered a barium swallow study, which revealed a normal radiographic motility pattern and transit of the barium column to the stomach. However, there was evidence of a structural abnormality appearing as a "shelf" impinging on the barium column at the level of the upper esophageal sphincter. The patient now presents to you for further evaluation and consideration for additional testing.

Vignettes 102-109: Answers

102. This is Chagas Disease. Chagas is a disorder that mimics achalasia. It is caused by infection with *Trypanosoma cruzi*, which is prevalent in Central and South America, and is spread by the reduviid bug vector (ie, the "kissing bug" that defecates in your eye while you are sleeping under a thatched roof hut—lovely). The *T. cruzi* parasite can disable ganglion cells throughout the GI tract and beyond, which leads to an achalasia-like picture of "megaesophagus," along with "megacolon" and cardiomegaly. The manometric findings can mimic achalasia (ie, aperistalsis, poor lower esophageal relaxation), with the exception of tonically elevated lower esophageal pressure—which is not a consistent finding in Chagas disease.

Here's the Point!

Dysphagia + Living Under a Thatched Roof Hut = Chagas Disease

103. This patient has paraneoplastic achalasia. This is a rare but classic and important presentation of lung cancer—most commonly small cell cancer. When this patient presented to our consult service as an inpatient, he reported a "nearly overnight" onset of bowel paralysis, like "a light switch." This is an important clue for paraneoplasia, since other processes (eg, malignant obstruction etc) tend to occur over time. Moreover, the simultaneous involvement of constipation and dysphagia is another clue for a more systemic process.

It is hard to invoke a single lesion that can simultaneously lead to dysphagia and constipation. It turns out that an epitope on small cell cancers mimics an epitope on the myenteric plexus. The so-called anti-Hu antibody forms against the epitope, and then affixes itself along the myenteric plexus throughout the GI tract. This can lead to paralysis of the esophagus (achalasia), stomach (gastroparesis), small intestine (intestinal pseudo-obstruction), and colon (colonic inertia). There may only be 1 segment of bowel affected, or many, as occurred in this case.

When our GI service interviewed the patient, we noticed that his voice was a little gravelly. We asked about this, and found out that it was a recent change—"my voice hasn't been that sharp lately," he said. He had a 50-pack-year history of smoking. The medicine service was surprised when our consult culminated in a request for a chest radiograph (Figure 103-1), which revealed a very subtle yet detectable haziness at the left upper lobe. A follow-up CT scan revealed a spiculated lesion which turned out to be lung cancer.

This is a great example of a GI consult that made a difference. Sometimes theory actually becomes reality, so learning this stuff clearly helps in "real life"—chance favors the prepared mind. In this instance the lung cancer was detected much earlier than it might have been otherwise. Had we not considered paraneoplastic achalasia, we would have probably detected typical achalasia changes on manometry (aperistalsis, elevated lower esophageal sphincter [LES] pressure, failure of LES relaxation with swallowing), and made a diagnosis of primary achalasia—all while the lung cancer was growing.

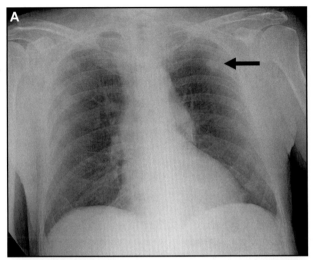

Figure 103-1. Chest film (A) and chest CT (B) of a former smoker with new-onset dysphagia and constipation. A chest x-ray was ordered because of concern for paraneoplastic bowel paralysis. The x-ray reveals a subtle haziness at the second rib on the left. The findings are subtle enough to have been missed had the pretest likelihood of malignancy not been brought to the radiologist's attention. The follow-up CT reveals a 1.5 x 1.8 cm stellate mass in the left posterior apical lobe, touching the pleura.

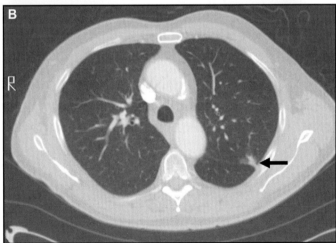

Here's the Point!

New-Onset Bowel Paralysis in a Smoker = Think Paraneoplasia

104. This is diffuse esophageal spasm (DES). DES is one of the "Big Four" motility abnormalities that you should know for the Board exam—the others being achalasia, nutcracker esophagus, and pelvic dyssynergia (see Vignette 24 for latter diagnosis). It is easy to confuse DES with nutcracker esophagus, since both are associated with high amplitude esophageal contractions in the setting of recurrent noncardiac chest pain. The difference between entities is that DES has nonpropagating simultaneous esophageal contractions, whereas nutcracker esophagus has propagating (albeit intense) esophageal contractions.

It is easy to forget which one is which—but just remember what a nutcracker does. In order for a nutcracker to crack a nut, it needs to transmit contractile forces downward along the nut, which allows for a much more efficient "crunch" than if the nut were simultaneously crushed from all sides. So, just like nutcracker esophagus, in which high-amplitude contractions (at least 180 mm Hg) travel down the esophagus in a peristaltic fashion, a nutcracker transmits high force contraction in a propagating manner along the length of the nut. Another difference between DES and nutcracker esophagus is that DES is very rare, whereas nutcracker esophagus is the most common manometric abnormality found in patients with a nonreflux esophageal etiology for chest pain. Both conditions can cause recurrent bouts of chest pain, with normal symptoms between flares.

In this case, the patient is unable to swallow anything during her bouts of chest pain, suggesting a nonpropagating motility disorder—ie, DES. If she were able to swallow, it would suggest nutcracker esophagus as a possible underlying diagnosis. The cause of DES remains a mystery. It probably has something to do with an imbalance between inhibitory and excitatory innervations of the esophagus. The diagnosis of DES ultimately relies on manometry, where spasm (at least 30 mm Hg pressure wave amplitude) is found in at least 20% of wet swallows.

In this case the manometry results were not provided, so you actually cannot be sure of the diagnosis until the manometric data are made available. The pressure waves in DES are simultaneous, often multi-peaked, and overlapping, as depicted in Figure 104-1.

This is similar to vigorous achalasia, in which there are overlapping high amplitude esophageal contractions, like with DES, but also with failure of the lower esophageal sphincter to relax. In this manner, vigorous achalasia is sort of a hybrid between classic achalasia and DES. In DES, the lower sphincter relaxes normally, and does not have high resting tone. In nutcracker esophagus, the pressure waves are high yet propagating, as depicted in Figure 104-2.

Treatment for both of these conditions is imperfect, but usually begins with a calcium channel blocker like diltiazem. Some use nitrates, although the data supporting this therapy are very limited. Others start with a PPI on the theory that flares are triggered by acid reflux. Finally, you could try something to modify visceral hypersensitivity (for the chest pain), such as a tricyclic antidepressant (eg, imipramine) or trazodone.

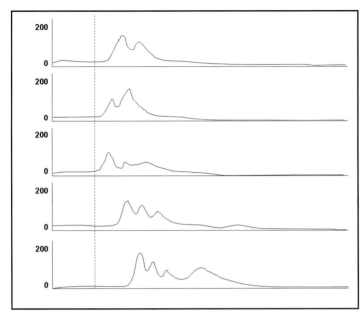

Figure 104-1. Manometric tracing in Diffuse Esophageal Spasm (DES). Note the high amplitude, simultaneous, non-peristaltic, multi-peaked contractions that occur after a wet swallow (denoted by dashed line).

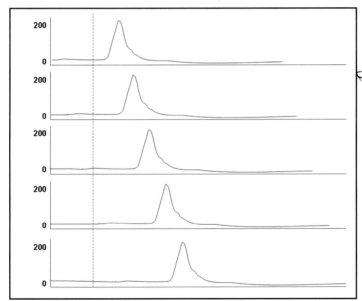

Figure 104-2. Manometric tracing in nutcracker esophagus. Note the very high amplitude contractions (>180 mm Hg) are peristaltic, in contrast to DES, in which they are overlapping and uncoordinated.

Here's the Point!

Nutcracker Esophagus = High Amplitude, Propogating Contractions
Diffuse Esophageal Spasm = High Amplitude, Non-Propagating

105. This is dermatomyositis. Dermatomyositis leads to dysphagia through weakness of the striated muscle in the proximal one-third of the esophagus. Characteristic symptoms include weakness in the proximal muscle groups, evidenced by difficulty standing from a seated position, or holding objects or weights overhead. The typical "heliotrope rash" of dermatomyositis appears as a violaceous ring around the eyes. The "shawl sign" appears as a discrete red patch behind the neck, like a red shawl. Gottron nodules appear on the knuckles. From a GI perspective, any redness on the eyes or neck in association with proximal muscle weakness and dysphagia = dermatomyositis. Steroids are the typical first line therapy for dermatomyositis-related dysphagia.

Here's the Point!

Red Eyes or Neck + Dysphagia = Think Dermatomyositis

106. This is the post polio syndrome. Patients with childhood polio can develop dysphagia up to 40 years after the original diagnosis. Although dysphagia is most common in patients with bulbar involvement at the time of the original infection, it may still occur, even in the absence of initial bulbar involvement.

Here's the Point!

Dysphagia years after polio = "Post Polio Syndrome"

107. This is systemic sclerosis. Systemic sclerosis leads to diffuse fibrosis of skin and smooth muscle tissue throughout the body. In the GI tract, this can lead to dysmotility across every segment of bowel, including the esophagus (aperistalsis from dysfunction of the distal two-thirds of the esophageal body), stomach (gastroparesis), small intestine (chronic pseudo-obstruction), and colon (colonic inertia). Up to 90% of patients with systemic sclerosis suffer from some form of bowel involvement, which can have severe clinical consequences.

"Megaduodenum" is a characteristic finding in which a nonobstructed, yet dilated, loop of duodenum is seen on barium studies of the foregut. There can be loops of dilated bowel throughout the jejunum and ileum as well. Bacterial overgrowth is common in these patients, which leads to bloating, diarrhea, abdominal pain, low B12 (from bacterial consumption), and high folate (byproduct of bacterial metabolism). Fat malabsorption can follow, leading to more diarrhea and weight loss.

Rarely, patients with systematic sclerosis can develop pneumatosis intestinalis, in which gas is trapped intramurally in the small or large intestine. This strange condition is also found, incidentally, in patients with chronic obstructive pulmonary disease. Its pathogenesis remains somewhat of a mystery, and is beyond the scope of this vignette.

In any event, the pneumatosis intestinalis lesion appears endoscopically as a submucosal rounded mass. Upon biopsy, the mass "deflates" and nearly disappears. I have seen this a few times, and every time it is initially perplexing and off-setting. But rest assured, if this happens to you, it is unlikely that you have actually perforated bowel. Instead, you have probably just popped a submucosal gas bubble.

Treatment principles of GI systemic sclerosis include repeated courses of antibiotics for bacterial overgrowth and promotility agents as tolerated. The esophageal symptoms can be alleviated with consuming smaller meals, avoiding late night meals, raising the head of the bed, and minimizing smoking, anticholinergic medications, and other substances that might reduce saliva production. Proton pump inhibitors are often necessary to combat erosive esophagitis—which could be severe, especially when there is concurrent esophageal and gastric dysmotility.

Here's the Point!

Dysphagia + Megaduodenum + Pneumatosis Intestinalis = Systemic Sclerosis

108. This is a cervical osteophyte. Cervical osteophytes are common in the elderly, and usually do not cause any problems at all. Rarely, when large, these bony lesions can protrude anteriorly into the posterior esophagus near or above the crycopharyngeus, or upper esophageal sphincter. When higher, they can protrude directly into the posterior pharyngeal constrictors, giving rise to solid-food dysphagia in the posterior pharynx upon transfer of the food bolus to the upper esophageal sphincter. This could give rise to a "globus like" sensation of fullness in the throat.

But unlike globus, there is a physical obstruction and true dysphagia to solids. Because osteophytes are so common, one must always bear in mind the potential for "true, true, and unrelated." That is, it is possible that a patient could have dysphagia, could have a cervical osteophyte on radiography, yet have some other underlying condition causing the dysphagia. However, if it is clear that the osteophyte is the culprit, then surgical excision is indicated assuming the dysphagia is sufficiently debilitating.

Here's the Point!

Dysphagia + Cervical Arthritis = Think Cervical Osteophyte

109. This is a cricopharyngeus bar. The cricopharyngeus is the upper esophageal sphincter (UES). The UES may become hypertrophic and form a "bar," which is radiographically detected as a smooth shelf impinging into the barium column at the level of the lower cervical spine. Bars occur as a normal variant in up to 10% to 15% of the population, and rarely lead to significant dysphagia. Endoscopy is a very unreliable test for detecting bars.

At best, endoscopy might reveal some "tightness" upon intubating the UES, but there are few reliable visual clues to establish the diagnosis with endoscopy alone. Esophageal manometry will reveal a high pressure zone in the upper esophagus, with normal pressures elsewhere. Bars are associated with various neurodegenerative conditions such as multiple sclerosis, amyotrophic lateral sclerosis, myasthenia gravis, stroke, and myopathies, although they usually occur in the absence of these conditions.

Although endoscopic dilation (with bougies or balloons) can be attempted, the definitive treatment for severe cases is a crycopharyngeal myotomy. It is important to emphasize, however, that not all bars cause symptoms, and not all cases of dysphagia in the setting of bars are actually from the bar itself. There have been cases of myotomy solving nothing—so it is not always definitive. In any event, surgery is not always a required solution, but in "true" cases of bar-induced dysphagia, it can be a definitive solution.

Here's the Point!

Dysphagia + Cervical "Shelf" on UGIS = Crycopharyngeus Bar

Vignette 110: Abrupt Vomiting

A 70-year-old man with a history of a large duodenal ulcer diagnosed 5 years ago, now presents to the emergency department with 12 hours of repeated vomiting. He had been in his usual state of health until 36 hours prior to admission, when he developed epigastric fullness shortly after eating a bag of prunes prior to bedtime. He could not sleep well, and felt an increasing epigastric pressure.

The next morning he felt "full and bloated," and was unable to tolerate any oral intake. This continued throughout the day, until he developed abrupt, large-volume, repeated vomiting. The vomitus was dark and nonbloody at first, but subsequently became tinged with blood after nearly 10 bouts of vomiting. He had similar symptoms 5 years prior to admission, when he was found to have a giant (3 cm) duodenal ulcer that was healed with PPI therapy.

Follow-up endoscopy from last year revealed a deformed duodenal bulb, but no residual ulcer disease. He reports no recent weight loss, melena, hematochezia, early satiety, dysphagia, or other GI alarm symptoms prior to the abrupt events of 36 hours ago.

Upon admission, he is found to be tachycardic and to have orthostatic hypotension that corrects rapidly with 1 L of normal saline. A nasogastric lavage retrieves more than 5 L of dark, nonbilious aspirate with coffee grounds.

His laboratories are significant as follows: Na=142; K=3.1; Cl=83; HCO3=32; BUN=50; Cr=1.3. The hemoglobin is normal at 13.2. His white cell count, platelet count, and liver tests are unremarkable.

▶ *What happened here?*

▶ *How does the electrolyte profile help make the diagnosis?*

▶ *What is the definitive treatment?*

Vignette 110: Answer

This is a gastric outlet obstruction from food plugging a deformed duodenal bulb. This patient presented to our emergency department at UCLA. Lo and behold, during the endoscopy we found a pitted prune lodged deep within a deformed duodenal bulb—just sitting there, barely digested or chewed. It took a bit of maneuvering with a Roth net, but we got it out. He woke up, and then we asked him if he likes prunes—he said yes. Then we told him he needs to chew his prunes. After the procedure he felt like a million bucks—he was ready to run right out the door.

Perhaps surprisingly, this story frequently repeats itself in other forms. More recently, we had a patient who abruptly plugged himself up after eating a big burrito. So it happens. The clue here is the history of a large duodenal ulcer and a deformed bulb. These deformed bulbs work—until they don't work. And often all it takes is a marble-sized, thick food product to stop up the works.

In this vignette the patient was fine until he ate a bunch of prunes, and then developed symptoms of acute gastric outlet obstruction, including nausea, fullness, bloating, anorexia, and repeated vomiting culminating in hematemesis. Indeed, we found a Mallory-Weiss tear at the gastroesophageal junction. The laboratories are classic for a gastric outlet obstruction. When the gastric outlet is blocked, acid accumulates and is vomited. This leads to a reduction in hydrogen and chloride ions.

Normally, for each hydrogen ion secreted into the gastric lumen by the parietal cell, there is 1 bicarbonate ion that drops into the gastric circulation, giving rise to the so-called "alkaline tide" that balances the acid wave in the stomach. The serum alkalinity is normally transient, because bicarbonate is taken up by the pancreas and deposited into the duodenum via pancreatic exocrine secretions. Under normal circumstances, hydrochloric acid (HCl) from the stomach travels into the duodenum where it immediately neutralizes the bicarbonate deposited by the pancreas. However, if there is a gastric outlet obstruction, the HCl cannot travel into the duodenum, and the bicarbonate dumped by the pancreas is not met by its neutralizing counterpart.

Thus, the bicarbonate goes unbuffered, and is ultimately reabsorbed into the body, leading to an alkalosis. This alkalosis leads to avid hydrogen reabsorption by the kidneys, and concomitant potassium dumping (through the H+/K+ exchange pump). In addition, there is dehydration, which leads to sodium preservation and further potassium dumping (through the Na+/K+ exchange pump). The net effect is a hypernatremic, hypokalemic, hypochloremic, metabolic alkalosis with an elevated BUN from dehydration.

If there is an underlying ulcer, then treatment consists of PPI therapy, avoiding NSAIDs, testing and treating for *H. pylori*, and, if warranted, ruling out hypersecretory states like ZES. If there is no inflammatory component, then patients should receive careful instruction about diet and careful chewing (eg, chew those prunes). If conservative dietary management is insufficient, then surgery is the definitive therapy, which requires reconstruction or removal of the deformed duodenal bulb.

Why might this be tested? Because the electrolyte profile is classic.

Here's the Point!

↑ Na + ↓ K + ↓ Cl + ↑ HC03 + ↑ BUN + Recurrent Vomiting =
Gastric Outlet Obstruction

Vignette 111: Pancreatic Cyst

A 68-year-old man undergoes a CT urogram to investigate a single episode of painless hematuria. The scan is normal, but reveals a vague heterogeneity on 1 cut of the pancreas. A repeat abdominal CT scan is performed, this time using a pancreatic protocol with intravenous contrast agent and thin pancreatic cuts. The scan reveals a fusiform cyst in the head of the pancreas, and a normal-caliber pancreatic duct.

A follow-up EUS reveals a side-branch cyst that is 1.5 cm in diameter. There is no evidence of septae, nodules, or thickening of the cyst lining. Fine needle aspiration of the lesion yields viscous fluid and a low CEA of 5. The amylase is over 10,000 units. The patient reports no abdominal pain, nausea, or vomiting.

A follow-up MRCP, performed 6 months later, confirms interval stability of the cyst size, and once again confirms the side-branch location without pancreatic duct dilation.

▶ *What is the most likely diagnosis?*

▶ *Is surgery warranted?*

Vignette 111: Answer

This is a side branch IPMN. The prevalence of pancreatic cysts, in general, has increased dramatically—a likely consequence of increased use and improved quality of abdominal imaging, coupled with the aging of the population. Some pancreatic cysts harbor malignancy, some are premalignant, and some have no malignant potential. Whereas IPMNs or mucinous cystic neoplasms (MCNs) are considered at increased risk for malignant transformation, other cysts, including serous adenomas or pseudocysts, have no known malignant potential. Moreover, it is often difficult to prognosticate. This clinical uncertainty is distressing to patients and their providers, who seek guidance in determining whether to do nothing, initiate invasive or noninvasive surveillance, or proceed directly to surgical resection—a seemingly draconian maneuver given the often low pretest likelihood for malignancy. Yet many patients are at risk for subsequent malignancy, so the clinical decision cannot be taken lightly.

In particular, the incidence of IPMNs has increased 5-fold in the last decade. At UCLA, one of the busiest pancreas centers in the country, IPMNs now comprise more than 40% of all pancreatic cyst resections performed. IPMNs can be divided into main duct (MD-IPMN) and branch duct (BD-IPMN) types depending on their anatomic relationship to the main pancreatic duct. Both are premalignant lesions filled with mucinous fluid, recognized histologically along a spectrum ranging from benign adenomas to invasive cancers. But MD-IPMN has a much higher malignant potential than BD-IPMN, which has a somewhat unclear malignant potential.

Because of the unpredictable natural history of these lesions, some argue in favor of surgical resection of advanced lesions, such as carcinoma in situ and invasive cancer, while continuing to survey patients with early lesions, such as adenomas. With current imaging techniques, including CT scanning, MRI, and EUS with pancreatic cyst fluid analysis, we are able to make the diagnosis of MD-IPMN and BD-IPMN with accuracy rates in the region of 80%. However, our ability to reliably predict the underlying histology or rate of malignant transformation is imperfect.

In light of this uncertainty, the Sendai Guidelines were developed to help establish whether and when to perform pancreaticoduodenectomy for these lesions. The guidelines state that any MD-IPMN should be resected, regardless of size or appearance. BD-IPMNs, as in this case, require a more nuanced approach, since many smaller lesions will never turn into cancer. The guidelines state that any BD-IPMN greater than 3 cm should be resected. Similarly, any lesion in association with recurrent upper abdominal pain should also be resected, since pain is a predictor of underlying malignancy. Lesions with nodules or thickening on EUS should also be resected, since those changes suggest early malignant transformation.

Cyst fluid can be very useful, as in this case. Data indicate that a CEA exceeding 192 is predictive of malignancy or imminent malignant transformation, thus prompting resection. The high amylase in this case only means that the cyst is in direct communication with the pancreatic duct, but does not necessarily portend a bad prognosis (since the lesion is not in the main pancreatic duct, only communicating with the duct along a side branch—an important distinction).

In this case, the cyst is relatively small, and there is no abdominal pain. The fluid CEA is low, there are no nodules or wall thickenings, and the lesion is stable in size over a 6-month period. Thus, according to guidelines, surgery is not warranted. The usual approach is to continue surveillance, either with repeated CT, MRI/MRCP, or EUS, at 6-12 month intervals. If the lesion is stable after several periods, then the interval can be extended. However, this part of the guideline is a moving target, so it shouldn't show up on a Board exam any time soon.

Why might this be tested? Because pancreatic cysts are extremely common, and their management is nuanced. Also, there are some clean clinical thresholds from the Sendai guidelines to memorize—always a good set-up for test questions.

Clinical Threshold Alert: If a suspected IPMN exceeds 3 cm in diameter, then resection is warranted. If the cyst fluid CEA exceeds 192, then the risk of malignancy is increased, and resection is warranted.

Here's the Point!

Cyst with Mucinous Content = IPMN until proven otherwise. Resect lesion if >3 cm, concurrent abdominal pain, nodules, high CEA on fluid aspirate, or if involving the main pancreatic duct.

Vignette 112: Diarrhea and Abdominal Pain in a Young Man

A 22-year-old man presents with 8 weeks of progressive abdominal pain, nausea, and nonbloody diarrhea. He is from Saudi Arabia, and recently traveled to the United States to study. He recalls the symptoms beginning shortly before arriving in the United States.

Since arriving, his symptoms have worsened. He has noticed lower extremity swelling around his ankles, and has involuntarily lost nearly 20 pounds. His appetite is poor.

Examination reveals a fever (T=100.8), signs of wasting, and lymphadenopathy in the cervical, axillary, and inguinal chains. A stool study is positive for qualitative fat, and his serum carotene is low. HIV is negative. His serum is positive for an alpha chain paraproteinemia. Upper endoscopy reveals a normal esophagus and stomach, and diffuse "cobblestoning" of the mucosa in the duodenum and proximal jejunum, as far as the scope can be passed. Biopsies reveal a dense lymphoplasmacytic infiltrate of the small intestinal mucosa.

▶ **What is the most likely diagnosis?**

Vignette 112: Answer

This is immunoproliferative small intestinal disease, or IPSID. IPSID is a subtype of gastric lymphoma, similar to marginal T-cell lymphoma (also known as MALT lymphoma). But unlike MALT and other typical forms of GI lymphoma, IPSID leads to the development of alpha heavy chain paraproteins. IPSID is almost exclusively found in the Middle East, and is more common in men than women. These are clues that might show up on a Board vignette, as depicted in this case.

The average age of onset is 25 years. IPSID is characterized clinically by abdominal pain, weight loss, lower extremity swelling, and malabsorption with attendant diarrhea. This is in contrast to non-IPSID GI lymphomas, which tend to occur later in life (30s to 40s on average), are not limited to the Middle East, and are not usually associated with a paraproteinemia, as with IPSID.

There are some other interesting features of this disorder. Namely, it is more common in areas of poor sanitation, suggesting a potential infectious etiology. In fact, it is associated with *Campylobacter jejuni* infection, and is usually treated first line with antibiotics directed against this organism (eg, ampicillin and metronidazole). Unfortunately, IPSID is an aggressive lymphoma, and is not usually cured with mere antibiotic therapy alone. Instead, it usually requires combination therapy with antibiotics, chemotherapy, and radiation therapy.

Why might this be tested? Because it is full of unique characteristics, including the Middle Eastern predominance, association with *C. jejuni*, expression of the alpha heavy chain paraproteinemia, and male predisposition—a perfect set-up for a Board question.

Here's the Point!

Young patient from Mediterranean region with dense lyphoplasmacytic infiltrate in the small intestine and a heavy chain paraproteinemia = IPSID

Vignette 113: Bloody Diarrhea After a Diverting Ileostomy

A 68-year-old man undergoes an urgent right hemi-colectomy and ileostomy for acute right-sided diverticultis complicated by a peridiverticular abscess. The surgeon plans to perform a subsequent reanastomosis of the ileum and remaining colon, but there is a delay in reoperating due to concurrent medical illnesses.

Three months after the operation, the patient develops rectal bleeding, tenesmus, left-sided abdominal pain, and a thick mucus discharge from his rectum. The output from his ileostomy is liquid, brown, and without blood. The patient reports no previous history of similar symptoms at any time prior to his operation.

The rectal effluent is sent for bacterial cultures, ova & parasites, and *C. difficile* toxin, all of which are negative. The symptoms persist, leading to evaluation by a gastroenterologist and subsequent colonoscopy, which reveals friable mucosa and diffuse apthous ulcerations, suggestive of diffuse colitis. Biopsies reveal preservation of the crypt architecture, but evidence of cryptitis with crypt abscesses, neutrophilic infiltrate in the lamina propria, and an increased density of lymphocytes and plasma cells.

▶ *What is the most likely diagnosis?*

▶ *What treatment should be initiated and why?*

Vignette 113: Answer

This is diversion colitis. As the name implies, diversion colitis occurs in segments of colon that have been diverted from the fecal stream as a consequence of surgery. The condition can develop within months of a colonic diversion, or may not arise until years later. It turns out that the fecal stream is important for colonic health. In particular, the stream includes abundant short-chain fatty acids (SCFAs), including acetate, n-butyrate, and propionate, among others. These SCFAs are critical for colonocyte metabolism, blood flow, and integrity. When SCFAs are absent, the colonocytes can lose their function, break down, and lead to a colitis-type picture.

Endoscopically, patients with diversion colitis can be indistinguishable from other forms of colitis, including inflammatory bowel disease, self-limited colitis, or infectious colitis. There may be apthous ulcers, which can mimic Crohn's Disease. The lack of chronic architectural distortion on biopsy, however, tends to argue against chronic IBD, where architectural changes are more common. However, the biopsy in diversion colitis shares other features of IBD, including crypt abscesses and cryptitis. There is often a mixed inflammatory infiltrate, including acute (neutrophils) and chronic (lymphocyte) components, along with plasma cells.

In this case, the lack of any preceding symptoms argues against IBD. The negative stool studies argue against an infection. Of course, *C. difficile* colitis is so prevalent, particularly in patients with recent hospitalization, that it should always be suspected—even if the initial *C. difficile* toxin is negative. However, the temporal association of the symptoms after surgery, coupled with the characteristic biopsy results, makes diversion colitis the most likely diagnosis.

Because the problem is lack of SCFAs, the natural treatment is to replenish this nutritional deficiency. This is most effectively accomplished with surgical restoration of luminal continuity, where possible. In patients who are not candidates for a reoperation, SCFA enemas can be very effective. The usual approach is to use a combination of sodium acetate, sodium n-butyrate, and sodium propionate. There is a fairly complex recipe to create the enema (need to balance pH and osmolality), and your local pharmacy should be familiar with how best to compound the mix—so those details should not be on an exam. But definitely be familiar with SCFA enemas in general.

Why might this be tested? Because it hits several areas all at once, including luminal GI, GI surgery, pathophysiology, and nutrition. And because there is a relatively simple and effective treatment in the form of SCFA enemas—a therapy that would never be provided if the diagnosis were consistently missed.

Here's the Point!

> Recurrent bloody diarrhea after ileostomy that improves with
> short chain fatty acid enemas = Diversion Colitis

Vignettes 114-120: Liver Masses

Liver masses. These can be tough to sort out, and they always show up—both on exams and, more importantly, in real life. So you need to know the basic approach to the radiographically identified liver mass. For each mini-vignette below, answer the question embedded within the text.

114. A 32-year-old woman on oral contraceptives develops severe, abrupt abdominal pain. An abdominal CT scan reveals a subcapsular mass in the liver and evidence of hemoperitoneum. What is the culprit lesion, and what happened here?

115. A 32-year-old woman on oral contraceptives undergoes an abdominal CT scan to evaluate recurrent abdominal pain. The scan reveals a 5 cm mass in the left lobe of the liver. On repeat triphasic CT scanning, the lesion is found to have a central scar with fibrous-appearing septae radiating from the scar like spokes of a wheel. The lesion is hypodense in the noncontrast phase and hyperdense during the hepatic arterial phase (Figure 115-01). A follow-up nuclear sulfur-colloid liver scan reveals marked uptake of the tracer. What is the diagnosis? Does this need to be surgically removed?

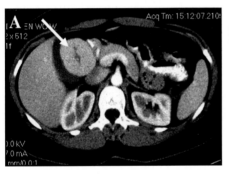

Figure 115-01. Arterial phase from triphasic CT scan of patient in Vignette 115. (Used with permission from Javier Casillas, MD, University of Miami, Miami, FL.)

116. A 65-year-old man with essential thrombocytosis is found to have an isolated, elevated ALP level. He undergoes abdominal CT which reveals multiple hypodense nodules in the right hepatic lobe. These are followed-up with a liver biopsy, which reveals regenerative nodules clustered around portal triads without fibrosis between the nodules. What is the diagnosis? What medication, often used for IBD, is also associated with this diagnosis?

117. A 52-year-old obese woman with diabetes undergoes abdominal ultrasound for evaluation of biliary colic. The ultrasound confirms multiple gallstones, but also reveals a 5 cm, irregular, hypoechoic lesion in the right hepatic lobe. Follow-up CT scanning reveals a hypodense, sharply demarcated mass. A subsequent MRI reveals increased intensity on T1 weighted images. The contour and architecture of the liver is not distorted in either imaging study despite presence of this lesion. What is the most likely diagnosis?

118. A 50-year-old man with alcoholic cirrhosis is found to have a 1 cm nodule in his left hepatic lobe on surveillance ultrasonography. The alfa-fetoprotein level is 10 ng/mL. The nodule enhances during the arterial vascular phase of a triphasic abdominal CT scan, and appears hypervascular upon gadolinium-enhanced MRI of the abdomen. What is the most likely diagnosis? Does this require a liver biopsy for confirmation?

119. A 50-year-old man with alcoholic cirrhosis is found to have a 2.5 cm nodule in his left hepatic lobe on surveillance ultrasonography. The alfa fetoprotein level is 450 ng/mL. The nodule enhances during the arterial vascular phase of a triphasic abdominal CT scan. MRI has not been performed. What is the most likely diagnosis? Is MRI necessary? Is biopsy necessary?

120. A 50-year-old man with alcoholic cirrhosis is found to have a 2.5 cm nodule in his left hepatic lobe on surveillance ultrasonography. The alfa fetoprotein level is 450 ng/mL. The nodule does not enhance during the arterial vascular phase of a triphasic abdominal CT scan, and does not light up with gadolinium-enhanced MRI. Is a biopsy necessary?

Vignettes 114-120: Answers

114. This is a ruptured hepatic adenoma. Hepatic adenomas are benign, but can be dangerous because they are often subcapsular, are highly vascular, and can spontaneously rupture. When they rupture, they can lead to massive exsanguination into the peritoneal cavity, as occurred here. In addition, hepatic adenomas can transform into cancer, so surgical resection is the treatment of choice.

They are strongly associated with oral contraception use, so the offending agent must be discontinued if the lesion is identified. They can regress after discontinuation of oral contraceptives, so there is some controversy about whether to remove smaller adenomas (ie, <5 cm) surgically or simply discontinue oral contraceptives and survey the lesion for evidence of regression. Because that is controversial, it is unlikely to be the subject of an exam question. But you certainly must know the diagnosis and its association with oral contraceptives. And for larger lesions (>5 cm), there is little debate that surgical resection is warranted even if oral contraceptives are discontinued.

115. This is focal nodular hyperplasia (FNH) of the liver. FNH is a relatively common and benign liver tumor that is much more common in women than men. Unlike hepatic adenomas, it is probably not caused by oral contraceptives, although this theory is sometimes floated around. In reality, nobody knows exactly what causes FNH, so I'll avoid the academic treatise on that topic for now.

In short, it is thought to result from a hyperplastic tissue response to abnormalities in vascular flow. Congenital arterial malformations have been implicated. The FNH lesion is characterized by hyperplastic regenerative nodules separated by fibrous septae. They classically have a central stellate scar with fibrous bands radiating circumferentially in a spoke-like pattern.

Patients with FNH are usually asymptomatic, but some have low grade abdominal discomfort. The characteristic scar can be seen on triphasic CT scanning. On CT, the lesion is hypodense in the noncontrast phase, but lights up upon arterial enhancement due to its vascular nature, as seen in Figure 115-01. Of note, the central scar does not light up with arterial enhancement, and remains hypodense, as seen in Figure 115-1 as well. A classic feature of this lesion is its affinity for sulfur-colloid uptake upon nuclear imaging. The lesion is benign, and surgery is not indicated.

116. This is NRH of the liver. NRH is a rare condition marked by regenerative nodules in the liver in the absence of fibrosis. Histologically, NRH appears as regenerative nodules clustered around portal triads without fibrosis between the nodules. It can lead to portal hypertension in extreme cases.

NRH is associated with a wide range of conditions and medications. Of the former, hypercoagulable states, myeloproliferative disorders, and lymphoproliferative disorders are among the most commonly associated conditions, as occurred here. Azathioprine has been associated with NRH as well, along with a host of other chemotherapeutic agents (eg, cyclophosphamide, chlorambucil, busulfan, bleomycin, carmustine, etc). The treatment is to either remove the offending agent, where possible, or treat the underlying associated condition (again, where possible).

117. This is a pseudomass from focal fatty infiltration. Fatty infiltration of the liver is common, particularly with the rising incidence of obesity, diabetes, and other components of the metabolic syndrome. On occasion, fatty deposition in the liver can be focal in nature—not diffuse, as is typically seen with nonalcoholic fatty liver disease. Focal fatty liver can mimic malignancy, and is classified radiographically as a "pseudomass" based on its sharply demarcated borders. Unlike a typical mass, however, focal fatty infiltration does not lead to a "mass effect" of compressed architecture surrounding the lesion or abnormalities in the contour of the liver. The focal fat is most commonly seen in vascular watersheds of the liver, such as the area around the falciform ligament, but can occur anywhere.

The lesions appear hyperechoic on ultrasonography. CT scanning may be inconclusive in distinguishing focal fat from an actual tumor or mass. The lesion is typically hypodense on CT. On MRI it lights up on T1 weighted images, which is characteristic of fat. In this case the most likely diagnosis is focal fatty liver given the risk factors (diabetes, obesity), the characteristic findings on 3 different imaging studies, and the lack of architectural distortion of the surrounding liver parenchyma. Biopsy would confirm fatty infiltration with "skip areas" of normal hepatic parenchyma around the fatty lesion.

118. This is most likely hepatocellular carcinoma (HCC), and does not require liver biopsy to confirm the diagnosis. Any liver nodule in a cirrhotic must be considered HCC until proven otherwise. The most commonly cited guidelines to determine the need for biopsy were developed by the European Association for the Study of Liver Diseases (EASL), so you should be familiar with the EASL recommendations. They are a bit complicated at first, but just learn them.

In sum, the guidelines state that any nodule greater than 2 cm in a cirrhotic should be considered HCC if 2 imaging studies (namely, a triphasic CT and a gadolinium-enhanced MRI) reveal a hypervascular lesion, regardless of alfa fetoprotein (AFP) levels. In this instance biopsy is not necessary, because the lesion exceeds 2 cm in size, and both the CT and MRI reveal a hypervascular lesion. So, even though the AFP is low, we must assume the patient has HCC, even without a biopsy.

Now, it gets a little more confusing as the permutations stack up—eg, high vs low AFP, 1 vs. 2 positive imaging studies, lesion larger vs smaller than 2 cm etc. The guidelines state that any lesion greater than 2 cm should still be considered HCC if the AFP exceeds 400 ng/mL and 1 of 2 imaging studies reveals a hypervascular lesion. Again, biopsy is not necessary to confirm HCC in this setting. The reluctance to perform biopsy, by the way, is because of the real risk of tumor seeding. So, in review, any cirrhotic with a liver nodule exceeding 2 cm should be diagnosed with HCC if the AFP exceeds 400 ng/mL and if 1 of 2 imaging tests are suggestive, or if 2 of 2 imaging tests are suggestive regardless of AFP levels.

Any other case typically requires a biopsy to confirm the histology. So there are 2 clinical thresholds to be aware of here: AFP of 400 ng/mL, and nodule size of 2 cm.

119. This is most likely HCC and does not require liver biopsy to confirm the diagnosis. Refer to the discussion above for the rationale. In particular, the AFP exceeds 400 ng/mL, and the CT reveals a hypervascular lesion. So a second imaging study (eg, MRI) is not warranted, nor is a biopsy necessary.

120. This is also most likely HCC, but it does require liver biopsy to confirm the diagnosis. Again, refer to the discussion above for the rationale. In this case the lesion is large (>2 cm) and the AFP is high, so the case seems open and shut. Yet the imaging studies do not reveal a hypervascular lesion. If only 1 of the 2 revealed characteristic findings, then biopsy would not be necessary and a presumptive diagnosis of HCC would be in order. However, the diagnosis is still in doubt, so a biopsy is necessary, even though there is a risk of tumor seeding from the procedure (if this really were an HCC). This can be confusing, so just study Table 120-1 to clarify the steps.

The table presents permutations of liver nodule size, AFP level, Triphasic CT scan results, and Gadolinium-Enhanced MRI scan results in patients with cirrhotics. Each row provides a permutation of these factors, and provides the action plan in the last column (eg, diagnose HCC empirically or proceed to biopsy).

Table 120-1

Nodule Size	AFP Level	Hypervascular on Triphasic CT?	Hypervascular on Gadolinium-Enhanced MRI	Diagnosis/Next Step
>2 cm	>400	Yes	Yes	HCC – No Biopsy
>2 cm	>400	Yes	No	HCC – No Biopsy
>2 cm	>400	No	Yes	HCC – No Biopsy
>2 cm	>400	No	No	Biopsy
>2 cm	<400	Yes	Yes	HCC – No Biopsy
>2 cm	<400	Yes	No	Biopsy
>2 cm	<400	No	Yes	Biopsy
>2 cm	<400	No	No	Biopsy (or monitor)
1-2 cm	>400	Yes	Yes	HCC – No Biopsy
1-2 cm	>400	Yes	No	Biopsy (tougher call!)
1-2 cm	>400	No	Yes	Biopsy (tougher call!)
1-2 cm	>400	No	No	Biopsy
1-2 cm	<400	Yes	Yes	Biopsy (but probably HCC)
1-2 cm	<400	Yes	No	Biopsy
1-2 cm	<400	No	Yes	Biopsy
1-2 cm	<400	No	No	Biopsy vs. surveillance
<1 cm	--	--	--	Surveillance imaging every 3 to 4 months

Vignettes 121-126: Dyspepsia

Dyspepsia refers to recurrent abdominal pain or discomfort in the epigastrium. It is common—very common. You should be familiar with the management principles of dyspepsia. Each mini-vignette, below, presents a patient with dyspepsia. For each one, decide whether the next step is to perform upper endoscopy, test for *H. pylori*, or prescribe a PPI.

121. A 28-year-old woman with reflux-predominant dyspepsia and no alarming signs or symptoms.

122. A 62-year-old man with reflux-predominant dyspepsia and no alarming signs or symptoms.

123. A 41-year-old woman with nonreflux predominant dyspepsia, described as meal-related pain in the upper abdomen, with a 10-pound weight loss over the last 6 weeks.

124. A 59-year-old man with nonreflux predominant dyspepsia, described as meal-related pain in the upper abdomen, without any alarming signs or symptoms.

125. A 33-year-old recent immigrant from China with nonreflux predominant dyspepsia, described as upper abdominal bloating with meals, without any alarming signs or symptoms.

126. A 33-year-old man with nonreflux predominant dyspepsia and *H. pylori* positivity, who has persistent symptoms despite a 10-day course of anti-*H. pylori* therapy. There are no alarming signs or symptoms.

Vignettes 121-126: Answers

Before answering the questions, it is worth reviewing dyspepsia in some depth. This is worthwhile because it is very common and often confusing. The discussion below follows the American College of Gastroenterology (ACG) 2005 guidelines regarding dyspepsia—a guideline widely employed by gastroenterologists, and among the most current evidence-based guidelines currently available.

Dyspepsia is defined as chronic or recurrent pain or discomfort centered in the upper abdomen. Discomfort is defined as a subjective negative feeling that is nonpainful, and can incorporate a variety of symptoms including early satiety, bloating, upper abdominal fullness, or nausea. Patients with predominant or frequent symptoms of heartburn or acid regurgitation should be considered to have gastroesophageal reflux disease (GERD) until proven otherwise. This is an important clinical distinction, because reflux-predominant symptoms imply underlying GERD, whereas nonreflux-predominant symptoms remain within the dyspepsia spectrum.

This is confusing to some providers, although it need not be. The confusion stems from the fact that GERD can indeed underlie nonreflux predominant dyspepsia. That is, GERD doesn't necessarily present with reflux predominant symptoms alone—it sometimes presents with epigastric pain or discomfort in the absence of reflux. Yet in the presence of reflux predominance, GERD is the leading diagnosis and the clinical picture is inconsistent with dyspepsia—a non-reflux-predominant syndrome.

Dyspepsia is divided into complicated and uncomplicated forms. Uncomplicated dyspepsia refers to symptoms in the absence of alarming features, including unintended weight loss, dysphagia, GI bleeding, iron deficiency anemia, guaiac positivity, physical evidence of malignancy (ie, abdominal masses, lymphadenopathy, etc), and other concerning signs or symptoms. Complicated dyspepsia refers to the presence of any of these alarming features.

The most common etiology for uncomplicated dyspepsia is "functional dyspepsia," which is sort of like IBS of the stomach (clearly an oversimplification). Functional dyspepsia accounts for roughly 60% of dyspepsia. Up to 25% of cases are due to underlying peptic ulcer disease, and 10% are from nonreflux-predominant GERD. Less than 1% of uncomplicated dyspepsia in the United States is from gastric malignancy. It can be difficult to distinguish these disorders on the basis of symptoms alone. Ulcer pain may be burning or gnawing in quality, but often the patient may simply have vague discomfort or cramping. Patients on concurrent aspirin or other nonsteroidal anti-inflammatory drugs have a higher pretest likelihood for peptic ulcer. Epigastric burning might be a sign of GERD, but also occurs with functional dyspepsia and peptic ulcer. Only the presence of "heartburn" or "regurgitation" is sufficiently specific for GERD. Other symptoms within the dyspepsia spectrum have poor sensitivity and specificity and cannot be relied upon to accurately discriminate between conditions.

A common dilemma in uninvestigated dyspepsia is whether or not to perform upper endoscopy early in the diagnostic evaluation. Because of the uncommon but important possibility that gastric cancer may be the underlying cause for dyspepsia, it is recommended that those patients who are at increased risk for developing gastric cancer undergo upper endoscopy. This includes patients over the age 55 or those who have "alarm features" which include: bleeding, anemia, unexplained weight loss >10% of body weight, progressive dysphagia, odyno-phagia, persistent vomiting, a family history of gastrointestinal cancer, previous esophagogastric malignancy, previous documented peptic ulcer, lymphade-nopathy or an abdominal mass. Patients fulfilling any of these criteria should undergo prompt upper endoscopy not only to rule out cancer, but to also to rule out peptic ulcer disease.

In patients younger than age 55 or with no alarm features, 2 main treatment strategies may be considered. The first is to test for *H. pylori* and treat if positive; if eradication is successful but symptoms persist, then a trial of acid suppression should be offered. The rationale behind this "test-and-treat" approach is that *H. pylori* eradication is highly effective in peptic ulcer disease, and has some (albeit modest) efficacy in functional dyspepsia. This strategy is most cost-effective in high prevalence populations (eg, recent immigrants from developing countries), where the prevalence of *H. pylori* typically exceeds 10%.

The most accurate noninvasive methods of testing for *H. pylori* are the urea breath test or the stool antigen test. If the patient tests positive, then the current treatment of choice is a combination of a PPI (standard dose twice daily) with amoxicillin (1 g twice daily) and clarithromycin (500 mg twice daily) adminis-tered for 7 to 10 days. Metronidazole (400 mg twice daily) may be substituted for amoxicillin in this regimen if the patient is allergic to penicillin.

The main disadvantage of the test-and-treat strategy is that the cure of *H. pylori* infection will only lead to symptom improvement in a minority of patients. However, there is evidence that test-and-treat is at least equivalent to prompt endoscopy in terms of outcomes. Several trials comparing the two have shown no differences in symptomatic outcomes or quality of life between the two groups at 1 year. Because of the cost of upper endoscopy, it is reasonable to pursue the test-and-treat strategy first in patients who are younger than 55 or without alarm features.

The second main treatment strategy for patients younger than 55 without alarm features is to first prescribe a course of antisecretory therapy empirically for 4 to 8 weeks. If the patient fails to respond or relapses rapidly after stopping the antisecretory therapy, then the test-and-treat approach should be applied before referral for upper endoscopy. This strategy is most cost effective in low prevalence populations where the pretest likelihood of underlying *H. pylori* is below 10% (eg, high socioeconomic areas, midwest region, etc, where the back-ground prevalence of ulcer or *H. pylori* is low). If an initial trial of acid suppres-sion fails and the patient is *H. pylori* negative, then it is reasonable to step up therapy by increasing the dose. While previous guidelines have recommended an empiric trial of H2-blockers for 6 to 8 weeks, recent studies reveal that PPI therapy has better symptomatic outcomes compared to H2-blockers in patients with dyspepsia.

In those patients who have failed both test-and-treat and the empiric trial of antisecretory therapy strategy, then the next step may be referral for upper endoscopy (if not already performed). However, endoscopy is not mandatory in patients without alarm features and the yield is low; therefore the decision to endoscope or not must be based on clinical judgment. Refer to Figure 121-1 for an overview of the dyspepsia algorithm described above.

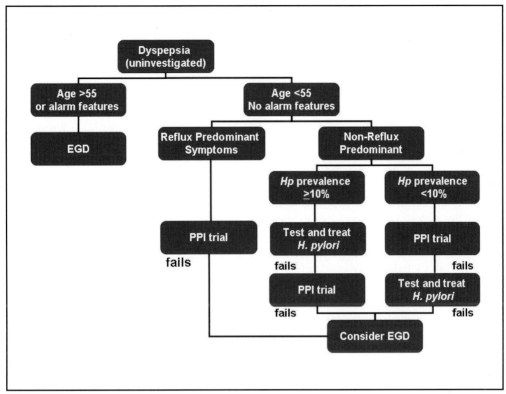

Figure 121-1. Algorithm for the management of uninvestigated, uncomplicated dyspepsia (adapted from Talley NJ, Vakil N, et al. Guidelines for the management of dyspepsia. *Amer J Gastroenterol.* 2005;100(10):2324-2337).

With this background, we can now answer the questions, as follows:

121. Start a PPI. In this instance, the patient has reflux-predominant dyspepsia, which implies underlying GERD. There is reason to believe that *H. pylori* eradication could potentially worsen—not improve—the symptoms of GERD in a patient like this, although it is somewhat debatable (see Vignettes 30 to 34 for details). In any event, this patient has GERD, is young, and has no alarming features, so antisecretory therapy is warranted to empirically treat likely GERD. Of course, an H2-blocker is perfectly warranted as well, but was not in the list of options for this question.

122. This patient probably has GERD, but needs to undergo endoscopy according to guidelines. Any patient over the age of 50 to 55 (depending on the guideline you read) needs endoscopy to screen for underlying malignancy or Barrett's esophagus (in the setting of GERD symptoms). This is controversial, but that is what the guidelines say. I could wax prolific about whether or not this is cost-effective, but for purposes of a Board exam, you should remain conservative and select endoscopy for anyone who is over the age of 55 with GERD or dyspepsia symptoms. That may or may not comport with actual real life practice, but the Boards do not necessarily correlate with real life.

123. This patient has dyspepsia. The most likely cause is functional dyspepsia by virtue of its population prevalence. However, the recent weight loss is an alarming symptom, and, assuming it is not intentional, should be taken seriously, even in a 41-year-old. The major concern, of course, is that she may have gastric cancer. Thus, endoscopy is the correct answer here.

124. This patient needs endoscopy. Although there are no alarming signs or symptoms, he is over 55 years old and therefore, according to guidelines, should undergo upper endoscopy to screen for malignancy even in the absence of alarming signs or symptoms.

125. This patient is young, has nonreflux predominant dyspepsia, and has no alarming features. Endoscopy is not warranted, and empiric PPI therapy is not a slam dunk because reflux is not the predominant feature. So the question is whether to employ *H. pylori* test-and-treat or empiric PPI therapy. As a recent immigrant from a high prevalence region for *H. pylori*, his pretest likelihood for the infection is high—surely higher than the 10% threshold cited in guidelines. So test-and-treat is the correct answer.

126. This patient is younger than 55, has nonreflux dyspepsia, and no alarming features. He failed *H. pylori* test-and-treat, so the next step, according to guidelines, is an empiric trial of PPI therapy—not endoscopy, as previous guidelines suggested.

Why might this be tested? Because dyspepsia is common, and its management lends itself to an algorithmic approach—a perfect setup for Board questions.

Clinical Threshold Alert: If a patient with nonreflux dyspepsia symptoms is older than 55 years, then endoscopy is warranted regardless of presence vs absence of alarm signs and symptoms. If the *H. pylori* prevalence in a community exceeds 10%, then *H. pylori* "test-and-treat" is the preferred first line approach for nonreflux predominant dyspepsia in patients without alarming features.

Vignette 127: GI Bleeding and Cutaneous Hemangiomas

A 31-year-old man presents to the emergency department after passing 4 black stools over the previous 12 hours. He feels "lightheaded" and "nauseous," but has not vomited. He complains of 1 week of progressive weakness, which culminated in the passage of black stools. He reports a history of iron deficiency anemia, but has not undergone endoscopic evaluation in the past for this diagnosis. He explains that family members also have developed anemia. He also reports a history of bowel obstructions, and explains that his intestines "get caught on themselves."

Previous medical records are not available. He does not use aspirin or non-steroidal anti-inflammatory drugs. There is no recent weight loss, fevers, chills, sweats, or other systemic symptoms. He reports no recent alcohol ingestion or retching. On physical exam he is alert and oriented. In the supine position, his pulse is 107 beats/min and his blood pressure is 101/65 mmHg. While standing his pulse increases to 119 beats/min, and his blood pressure drops to 91/52 mmHg. His abdomen is soft, nondistended, and nontender. There are no surgical scars. There are no stigmata of chronic liver disease. Rectal exam reveals black, tarry stool. There are several cutaneous hemangiomas scattered along the trunk, lips, and tongue. Labs include: Hgb=8.6; Platelets=395K; WBC Count=10.7; INR=1.0; Total Bilirubin=1.2; Creatinine=0.9.

▶ **What is the most likely diagnosis?**

▶ **What probably caused his previous small bowel obstructions?**

Vignette 127: Answer

This is Blue Rubber Bleb Nevus Syndrome (BRBNS). BRBNS is a rare condition marked by cutaneous and visceral cavernous hemangiomas. The visceral lesions often involve the GI tract, including the stomach, small intestine, and colon. BRBNS follows an autosomal dominant pattern of inheritance, although nonfamilial forms have been described.

Patients often present with iron deficiency anemia from slow bleeding, but may also present with large volume exsanguination, as occurred here. Gastric lesions are especially common and can bleed profusely. Small bowel lesions can serve as lead points for intussusception—the likely explanation for his previous bouts of small bowel obstruction.

If the lesions are localized, then they may be treated with surgical resection. But the lesions are more commonly diffuse, so surgical resection is usually not a tenable option. Conservative management with oral iron is typically the treatment of choice. Endoscopic therapy has not been widely reported because these highly vascular lesions are not well-suited for coagulation, and may be too large for clipping. Of note, there is another rare condition, called Klippel Trenaunay Weber Syndrome, marked by cutaneous and GI hemangiomas. This condition also features bone overgrowth, soft tissue hyperplasia, and varicose veins.

Why might this be tested? Because examiners love to make sure you know dermatological manifestations of GI diseases, and this is one of the classics (see Vignettes 9-16 for other classics). And everyone loves to say "Blue Rubber Bleb," so why not test on it?

Here's the Point!

Cavernous Hemangioma + GI Bleeding + History of Intussusception =
Blue Rubber Bleb Nevus Syndrome

Vignette 128: Intrahepatic Stones and Biliary Strictures

A 46-year-old man presents to the emergency department with acute-onset right-upper quadrant pain with radiation to the right shoulder. The patient is a recent immigrant from Hong Kong. His pain began 2 days prior to admission. It builds steadily, stays elevated for several hours, and wanes—but has not disappeared since beginning 2 days ago. One day prior to admission he became yellow, developed nausea, and vomited.

On the day of admission he developed chills and subjective fevers. He reports similar episodes on-and-off for the past 3 years, but has not sought treatment until now. He does not drink alcohol and does not use prescription medications or herbal supplements. There is no history of viral hepatitis. There is no recent weight loss.

On examination he has a fever of 101.4, BP of 110/80 without orthostatic hypotension, pulse of 110, respiratory rate of 16, and oxygen saturation of 98% on room air. He is jaundiced. There are no stigmata of chronic liver disease. The gallbladder is not palpable, and the Murphy's sign is negative. However, he is tender to palpation in the right upper quadrant. The liver edge is not palpable. There is no rebound or guarding.

Labs include: total bilirubin=12.8 (direct=9.1); AST=60; ALT=72; INR=1.1; albumin=3.3; ALP=620; WBC=16.2 (90% PMNs); Creatinine=1.4. An ultrasound in the emergency department reveals diffuse intra- and extrahepatic duct dilatation, along with innumerable stones in both the intra- and extrahepatic ducts. A subsequent ERCP is performed with direct cholangioscopic viewing of the ductal system (Figure 128-1).

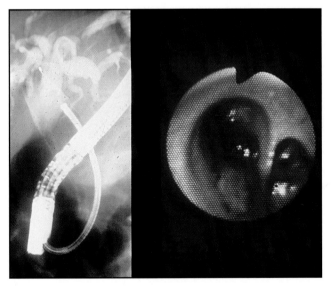

Figure 128-1. Left panel is cholangiogram from ERCP. Right panel is direct cholangioscopy of the intrahepatic ducts. (Used with permission from DiMarino AJ, Benjamin SB, eds. *Gastrointestinal Disease: An Endoscopic Approach.* Thorofare, NJ: SLACK Incorporated; 2002:1149.)

▶ **What is the most likely diagnosis?**

▶ **What are the short-term and long-term management steps?**

Vignette 128: Answer

This is recurrent pyogenic cholangiohepatitis, also known as Oriental cholangiohepatitis. This condition is strange, and a complete review of its pathogenesis and management is way beyond the scope of this book—namely because there is so much unknown about why this condition even occurs. The short story is that Oriental cholangiohepatitis (not a great term, by the way, but a long-used term that has become standard parlance) is almost exclusively seen in Southeast Asia—with a particularly high prevalence in rural areas of China, and in Hong Kong.

Its cause is unknown, and has been variably blamed on bacterial infections, parasitic infections, and abnormal biliary stasis. The condition is marked by the formation of innumerable pigment stones throughout both the intra- and extrahepatic biliary systems. The left hepatic system is classically affected for unclear reasons—possibly due to tighter angulations of the left vs right ductal takeoffs.

Patients typically present with bouts of acute cholangiohepatitis, marked by Charcot's Triad of right upper quadrant pain, jaundice, and fever. When severe, they can develop ascending cholangitis with Reynold's Pentad, which is Charcot's Triad with the additional features of hypotension and altered mental status. The bouts are usually recurrent and, over time, lead to severe stricturing from fibrosis of the ductal system. Intrahepatic abscesses may form, along with recurrent bouts of sepsis.

Management of acute attacks includes intravenous fluids and antibiotics, with attempts to remove as many stones as possible through ERCP. Figure 128-1 reveals intrahepatic stones on cholangiography, and black pigmented stones on cholangioscopy. ERCP can also be used to dilate the inevitable strictures that form with recurrent attacks. Unfortunately, ERCP alone is rarely adequate, and is often coupled with percutaneous t-tube drainage, or even surgical resection of affected hepatobiliary segments. Ursodeoxycholic acid (UDCA) is often used, but is probably of no real benefit for most patients. That is because UDCA does not effectively dissolve calcium bilirubinate pigment stones, in contrast to their efficacy for cholesterol stones. In patients where stone analysis reveals a cholesterol component, UDCA may be useful. But it should not be considered first line therapy for this complex disorder, which typically requires multi-modal approaches including endoscopic, radiographic, and surgical therapies.

Why might this be tested? Because this is a rare condition packed full of Board buzzwords and factlets (eg, intrahepatic pigment stones, left ductal system involvement, recurrent cholangitis in someone from Southeast Asia, etc).

Here's the Point!

Asian + Recurrent Pyogenic Cholangiohepatitis + Intra- and Extrahepatic Pigment Stone Disease + Diffuse Bile Duct Dilatations and Strictures = Recurrent Pyogenic Cholangiohepatitis ("Oriental" Cholangiopathy)

Vignette 129: Fever, Abdominal Pain, and a Skin Rash

You are consulted to evaluate an inpatient to assist with the diagnosis of recent onset abdominal pain. The patient is a 54-year-old Caucasian woman who recently traveled to Nepal. Two weeks after returning from her trip, she developed progressive chills, subjective fevers, and right lower quadrant abdominal pain. The fevers were initially low grade, but subsequently increased each day thereafter until they peaked at 103.2 on the day of hospital admission. There has been no diarrhea, bloody stools, or vomiting. The pain is constant and severe. She reports no previous abdominal pain of note, no joint or eye symptoms, and no family history of digestive disorders.

On exam she is febrile (temperature=101.4), has a pulse of 72, and a blood pressure of 90/62. There is no orthostatic hypotension. Skin exam reveals faint, diffuse, "salmon colored" macules across her trunk. She is not jaundiced, and there are no stigmata of chronic liver disease. She has marked tenderness in her right lower quadrant with voluntary guarding, but no rebound tenderness or involuntary guarding. Rectal exam reveals brown stool in the vault. A CT scan performed in the emergency department revealed thickening of the cecum and terminal ileum. Laboratories include: Hgb=10.1; WBC=16.2 (86% PMNs); platelets=320; amylase=30; lipase=28; ESR=14; CRP<1.0; AST=110; ALT=146; ALP=42; total bilirubin=1.9; INR=1.1; albumin=3.3.

▸ **What is the most likely diagnosis?**

▸ **How do the vital signs help establish the diagnosis?**

Vignette 129: Answer

This is typhoid fever from infection with either *Salmonella typhi* or *S. paratyphi*. Typhoid fever is a classic Board-type condition because it can so easily mimic other acute intraabdominal processes. Plus, it is one of the conditions that can affect the terminal ileum, and Board examiners love anything that can affect the terminal ileum.

Typhoid fever usually begins within 7 to 21 days after ingestion of the culprit organism. It is rare in the United States (although reported), and is most commonly contracted from ingestion of contaminated food or water in foreign countries (especially in those who neglected to get vaccinated for typhoid ahead of time). The prevalence of *S. typhi* and *S. paratyphi* is especially high in Nepal—a classic location for developing typhoid fever.

The condition usually begins with a complex of severe abdominal pain and "stepwise fevers," in which the fever curve follows a sort of step-like pattern of progressive elevations. Another unusual feature of the fever is a "temperature pulse dissociation," in which the heart rate is bradycardic in relation to the fever. In this case the pulse of 72 is quite low for such a high fever—even if this patient were an athlete. This is also seen with Leptospirosis, by the way, as described in Vignette 1.

The abdominal pain of typhoid fever can be severe, and is often in the right lower quadrant from underlying terminal ileitis or cecitis. In severe cases the bowel can perforate, leading to a surgical emergency. In the second week of the illness the patient may develop so-called "rose spots," which are faint salmon-colored macules across the trunk. Patients may also develop a hepatitis-like picture with elevated transaminases and bilirubin, as occurred here. The red herring on a Board exam would be Crohn's disease, which can also present with terminal ileitis and abdominal pain in the absence of bloody diarrhea.

In this case that diagnosis seems unlikely, as the symptoms began after traveling to a country endemic for the causal agent, there is temperature-pulse dissociation, the ESR and CRP are normal, and there are no classic IBD extraintestinal symptoms on review of systems. Treatment is with a quinolone, although drug-resistant strains are common so culture and sensitivity are mandatory.

Why might this be tested? Examiners love anything that may affect the terminal ileum, and this is one of the classics. This condition is also chock-a-block full of potential Board buzzwords, like "temperature pulse dissociation," "rose spots," abdominal pain and fevers after being in Nepal, etc. Finally, it affects both the intestines and the liver, so it can be "counted" in both bins as testmakers ensure sufficient coverage of all content frontiers. In short, it seems like a good condition to know about for the exam.

Here's the Point!

> "Stepwise" fever + Abdominal pain + Temperature-pulse dissociation + "Rose spots" on trunk and abdomen = Typhoid Fever

Vignettes 130-134: Crohn's Diarrhea

Below is a series of "mini-vignettes" in patients with Crohn's disease and diarrhea. For each patient, identify the most likely culprit for the diarrhea and its treatment.

130. A patient with Crohn's undergoes resection of 50 cm of TI for stricturing disease. He subsequently develops voluminous diarrhea.

131. Same as above, except 120 cm of TI is removed.

132. Patient with Crohn's colitis develops worsening of diarrhea after beginning therapy with a mesalamine (5-ASA) dimer.

133. Patient with Crohn's colitis develops severe diarrhea, fevers, and leukocytosis after starting metronidazole for perianal fistulizing disease.

134. Patient with fibrostenotic Crohn's disease limited to the small intestine develops progressive bloating, abdominal discomfort, and diarrhea in the setting of an elevated folate level and a depressed vitamin B12 level.

Vignettes 130-134: Answers

130. This is bile salt diarrhea. Bile salts are normally reabsorbed in the terminal ileum. Even minimal resection of the TI can affect bile salt resorption. As bile salts stay intraluminally, they pass into the colon in higher than normal concentrations. Once in the colon, bile salts irritate the colonic mucosa and lead to a secretory diarrhea. When up to 100 cm of TI is removed, bile salt dumping occurs and diarrhea may ensue. When more than 100 cm is removed, there is virtually no ability to resorb bile salts, so the salts become totally depleted—there is none left to even dump into the colon. In this case there is a fat malabsorption and steatorrhea. So, in both instances (<100 vs >100 cm resected) there is diarrhea, but the mechanism is different. When <100 cm is resected, the diarrhea is from a secretory diarrhea due to bile salt dumping. When >100 cm is resected, the diarrhea is from fat malabsorption. The former condition is treated with cholestyramine, and the latter with medium chain triglycerides.

131. This is fat malabsorption. See rationale above. Treatment is with a medium chain triglyceride.

132. This is likely 5-ASA-induced diarrhea. Although 5-ASA compounds are often used to treat colitis-related diarrhea, they can, themselves, induce diarrhea. In particular, the 5-ASA dimer products are most prone to cause diarrhea (up to 1 in 5 patients suffers this adverse event from 5-ASA dimers). They have fallen out of favor for just this reason.

133. This is likely *C. difficile* colitis. As a general principle, IBD flares should always prompt a search for underlying infection. In this case, the patient developed new-onset diarrhea after receiving metronidazole—a classic *C. difficile* culprit. *C. difficile* has become more and more prevalent, so it should always be high on the differential for anyone with diarrhea after antibiotics, IBD or no IBD.

134. This is small intestinal bacterial overgrowth (SIBO). Because SIBO has gained lots of attention in recent years, it is worth spending an extra moment to review the definition, associations, diagnostic testing strategies, and treatment of SIBO. SIBO is marked by an abnormal displacement of colonic type flora into the small intestine, including gram-negative organisms, enterococcus, and anaerobes. SIBO is classically associated with a range of conditions affecting small intestinal motility, structure, or immunity, including abdominal surgeries, diabetes, achlorhydria, scleroderma, ileocecal incompetence, and, as seen here, inflammatory bowel disease (especially when there is structuring). SIBO characteristically leads to the curious combination of low B12 and high folate. This occurs because the bacteria consume cobalamine (B12) and produce folate as a byproduct.

Because SIBO can lead to a range of bothersome symptoms and sequelae (diarrhea, constipation, bloating, gas, abdominal pain, cobalamine deficiency, malabsorption, etc), efforts have been made to develop accurate diagnostic tests to allow timely identification and treatment. The traditional gold standard for diagnosing SIBO is to perform a jejunal aspirate and culture the resulting fluid.

Whereas the jejunum normally has no more than 10^3 colony forming units (CFU) of colonic type bacteria in health, the concentration exceeds 10^5 in SIBO.

However, jejunal aspirates have been criticized because they may not reach areas that matter. Since bacterial migration begins distally, early forms of SIBO may not be detected if a jejunal aspirate is the only method employed for diagnosis. Moreover, stool DNA fingerprinting studies indicate that there are vast species of bacterial flora that are as yet undescribed, and thus most bacteria in the GI tract cannot be cultivated using conventional culture-based methods. Because cultures can only be limited to species that are known, jejunal aspirates are potentially limited by the extent of knowledge about active and currently measurable species.

Hydrogen breath testing (HBT) was developed as an alternative approach to diagnosing SIBO. Breath testing involves oral administration of a carbohydrate, such as lactulose or glucose, which is subsequently fermented upon exposure to colonic-type bacteria. This yields the production of hydrogen gas, which can be detected as a constituent in expired air. Since hydrogen gas is not endogenously produced in the absence of bacteria, the presence of any hydrogen gas in expired air implies carbohydrate fermentation by colonic-type bacteria. In health, hydrogen production does not typically rise before 90 minutes following carbohydrate ingestion. An earlier rise connotes proximal migration of colonic-type bacteria into the proximal small bowel. Similarly, a "double peak" suggests the presence of 2 populations of colonic-type bacteria: 1 in the small intestine, and 1 in the large intestine. Finally, a >20 part per million (ppm) rise by 180 minutes is also indicative of SIBO.

Lactulose hydrogen breath testing (LHBT), in particular, has been advocated as the optimal method, since lactulose is not absorbed and thus remains eligible for fermentation in the distal small bowel. In contrast, glucose can be absorbed proximally, so distal SIBO may not be detected as readily with this agent. Importantly, HBT does not require knowledge of the full taxonomy of bowel flora, as is required of jejunal aspirate and cultures, in order to be fully predictive. Treatment of SIBO is typically with a single 7 to 10 day course of an appropriate antibiotic, such as tetracycline, neomycin, norfloxaxin, or rifaximin, among others. Of course, where possible, the underlying condition should be treated as well. In this case, there is stasis related to small intestinal strictures, so surgery might ultimately be warranted.

Vignette 135: Chronic Diarrhea

A 22-year-old graduate student presents with 6 months of watery diarrhea. She reports having BMs 3 to 4 times daily. She describes bloating and visible distension accompanying the diarrhea, but no abdominal pain. Bowel movements do not improve the bloating. There is no blood in her BMs. She does not report incontinence. The diarrhea does not wake her from sleep—it is strictly problematic during the day. The symptoms occur daily, although she recalls an improvement on the day she fasted for a religious holiday.

She reports no weight loss, nausea, vomiting, fevers, chills, or sweats. She has not traveled recently, and has not been exposed to sick contacts. She recently tested negative for HIV—a test she performed for asymptomatic screening. She has not received antibiotics for more than 2 years. Although she reports being under some stress from school work, she does not link episodes of stress to her diarrhea. There is no family history of IBD, IBS, celiac sprue, or other digestive disorders. She takes no medications or herbal supplements.

Her examination fails to identify pertinent positives. Laboratories include a normal blood count, electrolytes, TSH, serum carotene, and anti tissue transglutaminase IgA. Stool electrolytes are measured, as follows: sodium=15, potassium=30. The stool pH is 4.

▶ *What is the diagnosis?*

▶ *What additional information should you obtain from her history?*

Vignette 135: Answer

This is osmotic diarrhea from carbohydrate malabsorption. Although stool anion gaps are rarely used in clinical practice, they are Board review favorites. And, I must admit, I still use the stool anion gap from time to time in clinic, and sometimes find it to be extremely useful. So it is probably worth remembering how to interpret the stool anion gap.

The idea is that the gap can help you distinguish osmotic from secretory diarrhea. Of course, you can often distinguish the two from history alone. In this case, the improvement with fasting argues in favor of an osmotic diarrhea, suggesting that unabsorbed osmoles in the diet are contributing to the diarrhea. Secretory diarrhea, in contrast, does not typically improve with fasting. Also, osmotic diarrhea often disappears at night, whereas secretory diarrhea can continue throughout the night. However, these features are often unreliable and inconsistent, so it is sometimes worth confirming one way or the other with an objective test—that is where the stool anion gap steps in.

The gap is calculated with the following formula: 290-2(Na+K), where the N+ and K+ are the stool measurements, not the serum measurements. When there are unmeasured osmoles, as occurs with carbohydrate malabsorption, there are relatively fewer measured osmoles (ie, Na+ and K+), so the 2(Na+K) term tends to be low, and the gap tends to be high. In contrast, with a secretory diarrhea there is high intraluminal Na+ and K+, so the 2(Na+K) term is high, and the gap is low. When the gap falls below 50 mOsm/kg, the diagnosis is secretory diarrhea. In contrast, when the gap exceeds this threshold, the diarrhea is more likely to be osmotic. In this case, the gap is 290-2(15+30)=200. Thus, the gap exceeds 50, and the diagnosis is most likely an osmotic diarrhea.

However, this is not enough information to confirm carbohydrate malabsorption as the root cause, as other noncarbohydrate ingestions (eg, laxative abuse with magnesium compounds) can produce the same stool anion gap. The two can be distinguished by checking the stool pH. When the pH falls below 5, it suggests that intraluminal carbohydrates have been fermented by colonic bacteria, leading to the liberation of short chain fatty acids and a low stool pH.

This is what happened here. So the next step is to dig back into the history and ask about dairy intolerance as a screen for lactose intolerance (if not already done as part of a complete history), a chewing gum habit (classic but rare cause of chronic diarrhea from sorbitol), ingestion of food additives or high sugar content (fructose, sucrose), or abuse of sugar-containing osmotic laxatives (eg, sorbitol, lactulose). A hydrogen breath test can be used to screen for specific sugar intolerances, and there are specific tests available for laxatives. Refer to Figure 135-1 for a review of these diagnostic steps.

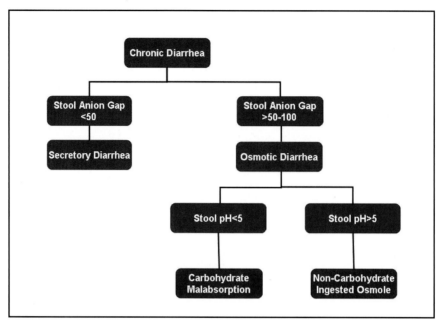

Figure 135-1. Algorithm for distinguishing secretory from osmotic diarrhea using the stool anion gap. Once osmotic diarrhea is identified, the stool pH can further distinguish carbohydrate malabsorption from ingestion of noncarbohydrate osmoles.

Why might this be tested? Because this relies on some basic memorization, but also requires that you combine rote numerical results with an understanding of the patient history. Also, chronic diarrhea, in general, is an important topic to know for the Boards.

Clinical Threshold Alert: If the stool anion gap is below 50, then the diagnosis is secretory diarrhea. If the threshold is above 50 (or 100, depending on who you talk to), then the diagnosis is osmotic diarrhea. In osmotic diarrhea, if the stool pH falls below 5, then the diagnosis is carbohydrate malabsorption. If it exceeds 5, then there is ingestion of a non-carbohydrate osmole.

Here's the Point!

Chronic diarrhea with stool anion gap >100 and pH<5 =
Carbohydrate Malabsorption

Vignette 136: Fear of Eating

A 28-year-old woman is referred to you for recurrent bouts of epigastric pain. The pain is always postprandial—typically within minutes of food ingestion. It lasts for several minutes and then improves. There are no symptoms between meals. The pain is severe, and she now has developed a progressive fear of eating, to the point of unintentionally losing 30 pounds over the last 3 months. She is often nauseous with the bouts of epigastric pain, but she does not vomit. There is no diarrhea, melena, or hematochezia. There is no history of hypertension, diabetes, or obesity. Examination reveals a bruit over the epigastrium. The patient is thin, and the abdominal aorta is palpable. However, there is no lateral expansion of the abdominal aorta evident on palpation. Abdominal ultrasound is negative.

▶ **What is the most likely diagnosis?**

▶ **What is the next diagnostic step to confirm this diagnosis?**

Vignette 136: Answer

This is median arcuate ligament syndrome, or celiac artery compression syndrome. Median arcuate ligament syndrome is a rare condition marked by abnormal compression of the celiac trunk by the median arcuate ligament, a fibrous structure that normally passes near—but not directly across—the celiac trunk. When the celiac trunk is compressed there is relative ischemia to the foregut, particularly when demand is highest after a meal.

Sitophobia describes fear of eating, and is a nearly pathognomonic symptom of GI vascular insufficiency. Of course, other conditions can cause fear of eating (say, a peptic ulcer), but big-time sitophobia within minutes of eating is usually not from a mere luminal ulcer. In any event, median arcuate ligament syndrome presents clinically with postprandial pain, sitophobia, weight loss, and (sometimes) an epigastric bruit, as occurred here.

The physical examination in this case is not consistent with an abdominal aortic aneurysm, which can also cause a bruit. Moreover, a triple-A should not cause postprandial pain and sitophobia. It is usually asymptomatic until it finally ruptures. The diagnosis of median arcuate ligament syndrome ultimately relies on characteristic imaging with angiography, including CT, MR, or standard radiographic angiography. There may be a concave indentation of the celiac trunk, and paradoxical flow with breathing—radiographic features that you would not be expected to really know, but that might help fill out the full picture in a patient like this.

Treatment is with surgical release of the median arcuate ligament. Unfortunately, it does not always provide relief, but that is another story.

Why might this be tested? Because these patients can be easily missed for years. The condition is rare, but you should always keep vascular etiologies in mind. Plus, you should be sure to program "vascular problem" into your brain whenever you hear about true sitophobia.

Here's the Point!

> **Sitophobia + Weight Loss + Postprandial Epigastric Pain + Epigastric Bruit = Median Arcuate Ligament Syndrome**

Vignettes 137-149: Pathology Buzzwords

You are probably not a pathologist. But for purposes of the Board exam, it is important to know a slew of pathology buzzwords to help navigate through many of the questions. This collection of mini-vignettes provides a set of classic pathology buzzwords with minimal surrounding information. The buzzword alone may be enough to get the diagnosis. Read each vignette, and then make the diagnosis.

137. A patient with cholestasis has a liver biopsy revealing a "florid duct lesion" marked by bile duct destruction, "ductopenia," and granulomas.

138. A patient with elevated transaminases and an elevated gamma globulin has interface hepatitis with a plasma cell infiltrate and lobular inflammation on liver biopsy.

139. A patient with recurrent infections, now with chronic diarrhea, undergoes small bowel biopsy, which reveals giardia in the absence of plasma cells in the lamina propria along with innumerable lymphoid nodules.

140. A patient with elevated transaminases has PAS-positive diatase resistant globules in hepatocytes on liver biopsy.

141. A patient on chronic therapy with a PPI has multiple gastric polyps with cystic dilatations on biopsy.

142. A patient with thickened gastric folds and a low albumin has foveolar hyperplasia on biopsy.

143. A former intravenous drug user is referred to you for persistently elevated liver enzymes (AST/ALT 3x ULN) and transferrin saturation (85%). Recent liver biopsy revealed presence of hemosiderin in Kupffer cells, but not in hepatocytes.

144. A 22-year-old with recurrent abdominal pain undergoes upper endoscopy which reveals focal patches of erythema. These reveal *H. pylori* negative. His ESR and CRP are elevated.

145. An elderly patient is found to have mucosal-based pearly nodules scattered throughout his esophagus. Biopsy reveals enlarged, mature squamous cells with glycogen-rich cytoplasm.

146. A patient undergoes endoscopy for reflux symptoms. There is no evidence of erosive esophagitis. Biopsy of normal-appearing mucosa 5 cm above the gastroesophageal junction reveals lengthening of the vascular pegs, epithelial hyperplasia, wide intercellular spaces, and 10 eosinophils/hpf. There are no abnormalities found at higher levels in the esophagus.

147. A patient with odynophagia has esophageal ulcers with "owl's eye" inclusions on biopsy.

148. During a drawn-out, tortuous, difficult colonoscopy, white patches are found in the ascending colon suggestive of leukoplakia. Biopsy reveals clear spaces in the mucosa and submucosa suggestive of fat cells—but without nuclei.

149. A young patient with vitiligo and premature gray hair undergoes endoscopy, which reveals prominent submucosal vessels and multiple erythematous nodules. Biopsy reveals increased endocrine cells throughout the body of the stomach, and biopsy of the nodules reveals nests of enterochromaffin-like (ECL) cells.

Vignettes 137-149: Answers

137. This is primary biliary cirrhosis (PBC). PBC is a progressive, destructive disease that decimates the bile ducts over time. When the disease becomes advanced, it produces a so-called "florid duct lesion" marked by bile duct destruction, a severe lymphoplasmacytic infiltrate in the portal tracts, and granulomas. Primary sclerosing cholangitis (PSC) can produce a similar appearance, but is not associated with granulomas. The classic feature of PSC is a fibrous obliterative cholangitis that looks like "onion skinning" around the bile ducts. Both PBC and PSC can lead to "ductopenia," or a lack of bile ducts altogether in the burnt out stage.

Here's the Point!

> **High ALP + Florid Duct Lesion + Granulomas = PBC**
> **High ALP + Florid Duct Lesion + Onion Skinning = PSC**

138. This is autoimmune hepatitis (AIH). AIH is classically associated with elevated transaminases in association with elevated gamma globulin levels. Characteristic histologic changes include interface hepatitis with a plasma cell infiltrate. In particular, the limiting plate of the portal tract is invaded by the infiltrating plasma cells, which, in turn, extend into the acini.

Here's the Point!

> **Interface hepatitis + plasma cell infiltrate = Autoimmune Hepatitis**

139. This is chronic variable immunodeficiency (CVID). CVID is among the most common forms of antibody deficiency, and is characterized by impaired B cell function and a low total IgG level. It classically presents with recurrent infections, most notably giardiasis. Normally, patients with giardiasis have a pronounced plasma cell infiltrate in the lamina propria in response to the organism. An absence of plasma cells in the lamina propria is highly suggestive of CVID. Endoscopically, patients with CVID often have innumerable mucosal-based nodules in the small intestine. Upon biopsy, these are confirmed to be lymphoid nodules.

Here's the Point!

> **Giardiasis + NO Plasma Cells = Chronic Variable Immunodeficiency**

140. This is alpha-1 antitrypsin (A1AT) deficiency. Refer to Vignette 27 for details.

141. This is fundic gland polyposis. Patients on chronic PPI therapy are prone to develop these gastric polyps, which are characterized by cystic dilatations of the oxyntic gland mucosa with attenuation of the parietal cells, chief cells, and mucous neck cells. As the name implies, fundic gland polyps are predominantly in the fundus, and are rare in the antrum (where oxyntic gland mucosa is not generally found). These polyps can be sporadic or familial. The sporadic type often arises from beta-catenin gene mutations and rarely leads to dysplasia or malignancy. They are considered to be benign and there is no specific treatment. The familial type can be seen in FAP, and are associated with the adenomatous polyposis coli (APC) gene on chromosome 5. See Vignette 150 for more information about FAP in general. The familial type fundic gland polyps often do contain dysplasia (around 25% of the time in some case series), so they need to be monitored and removed once dysplasia is detected. The details for how and when to perform surveillance remain somewhat controversial and unclear, so that should not be the topic of a Board question. But you should certainly know that fundic gland polyps in FAP are different, both genetically and pathologically, compared to the sporadic fundic gland polyps that tend to arise in the setting of PPI therapy. Finally, it gets a little more complicated than this, because even the sporadic type (ie, non-syndromic) fundic gland polyps can occasionally develop dysplasia (around 3% in some case series). Recently, investigators have found that the dysplasia in the sporadic polyps is also associated with APC alterations, even in the absence of underlying FAP. So there might be some mixing and matching here. The implication is that there might be a role for APC and beta-catenin testing in patients found to have fundic gland polyps, but the jury is out regarding exactly when and how to do this. For purposes of Board review, I'd at least know about the different types of fundic gland polyps, the varying risk of dysplasia in sporadic vs familial type polyps, and the relationship between dysplasia risk and APC vs beta-catenin genetic mutations.

> ### Here's the Point!
>
> **PPI Therapy + Gastric Polyps with Cystic Dilations = Fundic Gland Polyposis**

142. This is Menetrier's Disease. See Vignette 26 for details.

143. This is hemosiderosis, probably from underlying chronic viral hepatitis. The key here is to distinguish hemochromatosis from hemosiderosis. The former leads to iron deposition in the hepatocytes, and the latter leads to iron deposition in the Kupffer cells, which are the macrophages of the liver. Both can be associated with an elevated transferrin saturation. Hemochromatosis may lead to transaminases elevations, but hemosiderosis, in and of itself, is less likely to cause transaminases to rise 3x the upper limit of normal, as occurred here. So we need to posit an underlying condition that can lead to both hemosiderosis and transaminemia. There are 3 common conditions that fit this bill: chronic viral hepatitis, nonalcoholic fatty liver disease (NAFLD), and alcoholic liver disease. This former IV drug user is at risk for viral hepatitis, in particular, so that should be high on the differential diagnosis.

Here's the Point!

Iron in hepatocytes = Hemochromatosis
Iron in Kuppfer Cells = Hemosiderosis

144. This is gastric Crohn's disease. Crohn's can affect the entire GI tract, from mouth to anus. In the stomach, Crohn's can present with a characteristic focal non-*H. pylori* gastritis. The patient's age, history of recurrent abdominal pain, and elevated ESR/CRP raise suspicion for underlying Crohn's disease. The finding of focal non-*H. pylori* gastritis does not necessarily cinch the diagnosis, but makes it very likely.

Here's the Point!

Focal Non-*H. pylori* Gastritis = Think Crohn's Disease

145. This is glycogenic acanthosis of the esophagus. These lesions are very common in the elderly. They are benign. They can be confused for esophageal candidiasis, so if there is any doubt, then biopsy can confirm the diagnosis by revealing enlarged squamous cells with glycogen-rich cytoplasm. There should be no hyphal forms.

Here's the Point!

Elderly + White Papules in Esophagus + No Hyphal Forms =
Glycogenic Acanthosis

146. This is acid reflux disease. It is important to know the basic histological footprints of chronic acid damage. In this case, there is no erosive esophagitis, but there is nonetheless evidence of chronic reflux disease. This is classified as nonerosive reflux disease, or "NERD." There are 4 cardinal features: (1) lengthening of the vascular pegs (also called "rete pegs"); (2) hyperplasia of the epithelial surface; (3) wide intercellular spaces; and (4) an inflammatory infiltrate, including eosinophils. The eosinophilic infiltrate is not at the level of eosinophilic esophagitis, which is usually above 15 to 25 per high power field. The lack of findings higher up in the esophagus also argues against eosinophilic esophagitis.

147. This is CMV esophagitis. CMV esophagitis is characterized by elongated, large, and often serpiginous ulcers in the esophagus. The ulcers can be deep, and may have an undermined sharp border. CMV tends to live in and around blood vessels, so they are best found at the base of ulcers. Biopsy reveals inclusions that appear like owl's eyes. In contrast, HSV esophagitis is characterized by smaller but more plentiful ulcers that look like little round volcanoes with raised borders with a central exudate (ie, the lava). HSV is a sort of garbage dweller that sits along the rim of the ulcer. So CMV is best found at the center (<u>C</u>MV=<u>C</u>enter) and HSV at the rim. As an aside, if you find a patient with CMV-related GI disease, be sure to check the retinae for CMV retinitis, since it is present in around 10% to 20% of patients with CMV involvement of the digestive tract.

Figure 147-1. A) Cytomegalovirus esophagitis. B) Herpes simplex virus. (Courtesy of Wilfred Weinstein, MD, David Geffen School of Medicine at UCLA.)

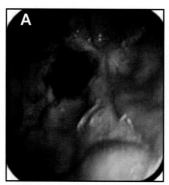
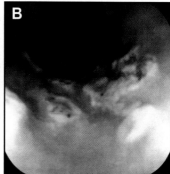

Here's the Point!

Know Table 147-1

Table 147-1		
COMPARISON OF CMV AND HSV ESOPHAGITIS		
Feature	*CMV Esophagitis*	*HSV Esophagitis*
Number of ulcers	Few	Multiple
Appearance of ulcers	Long, serpiginous, deep, with undermined edges	Round, small, superficial, "volcano-like"
Location of ulcers	Usually middle to distal third of esophagus	May be throughout the entire length of esophagus
Odynophagia	Can be severe	Often less severe than CMV (though not always)
Where to biopsy for organism	Center of ulcer	Edge of ulcer
Microscopic appearance	"Owl's eye" inclusion bodies	"Ground glass" nuclei; eosinophilic "Cowdry Bodies"; multinucleated giant cells
Treatment	Ganciclovir first line, foscarnet second line	Acyclovir

148. This is pseudolipomatosis from insufflation artifact. Although rare, intraluminal air can occasionally dissect into the mucosal and submucosal tissue planes of the colon. This usually occurs during long, drawn out colonoscopy where an inordinate amount of air is employed to compensate for a technically difficult procedure. The insufflation artifact can appear as white patches like leukoplakia on macroscopic appearance. Microscopically, there are clear spaces from the air itself. This can mimic fat cells, except the lack of nuclei confirms that the spaces are filled with air and not individual cells. The lesion is benign and resolves spontaneously.

Here's the Point!

Technically challenging colonoscopy + Focal white patches with clear spaces on biopsy = Pseudolipomatosis

149. This is pernicious anemia with atrophic gastritis and carcinoids. The history of vitiligo is a tip-off, because autoimmune conditions are often comorbid in pernicious anemia. Also, patients with pernicious anemia may develop premature graying of the hair, as occurred here. The endoscopy suggests atrophic gastritis, as the prominent vasculature indicates an attenuated mucosal surface. Although not described in this vignette, loss of rugae is also endoscopically characteristic of atrophic gastritis. The biopsy reveals enterochromaffin-like (ECL) cells throughout the mucosa, along with nests of ECL cells, suggestive of carcinoids, which occur in pernicious anemia as a consequence of hypergastrinemia. See Vignettes 29-33 for a review of gastrin physiology and why gastrin is elevated in pernicious anemia.

Here's the Point!

Pernicious Anemia + Gastric Bumps with ECL Cells = Carcinoids

Vignettes 150-155: Hereditary Colorectal Cancer Buzzword Associations

Board review is a great time to test your knowledge of hereditary colorectal cancer syndromes. These syndromes make for great test question fodder, because they have stereotyped presentations and eminently testable clinical associations.

Below is a collection of comorbid conditions that travel along with different hereditary syndromes. These are classic Board review buzzwords. For each buzzword listed below, identify the hereditary colorectal cancer syndrome that is associated with that condition.

150. Mandibular osteoma

151. Ureteral cancer

152. Facial angiofibromas (adenoma sebaceum)

153. Medulloblastoma

154. Trichilemmoma

155. Sertoli cell testicular tumors

Vignettes 150-155: Answers

150. This is Gardner's Syndrome, a variant of FAP. Before reviewing Gardner's Syndrome, it is first important to review FAP. FAP is an autosomal dominant condition that arises from a germline mutation in the adenomatous polyposis coli (APC) gene on chromosome 5.

Patients with FAP develop hundreds of adenomatous polyps that carpet the colon. Cancer is inevitable. The average age of polyp formation is 16 years, and the average age of cancer formation is 39 years. This has obvious surveillance and colectomy implications, since the progress to cancer is rapid, inexorable, and without exception. At-risk family members must begin annual screening with flexible sigmoidoscopy starting at puberty. If there is no evidence of advanced polyposis by age 40, then the surveillance interval can be lengthened to every 3 years.

Once polyposis occurs, patients should be referred for prophylactic colectomy. Of note, FAP is associated with a wide range of extracolonic manifestations as well. When there are extracolonic findings, the condition is called Gardner's Syndrome. Extracolonic findings in Gardner's include mandibular and skull osteomas (buzzword in this vignette), desmoid tumors, lipomas, fibromas, epidermoid cysts, and sebaceous cysts. Other classic associations include supernumerary teeth, mesenteric fibromatosis, and congenital hypertrophy of the retinal pigmentation epithelium.

As FAP and Gardner patients live longer with timely prophylactic colectomy, we have started to see the second wave of GI malignancies, chief among them duodenal and ampullary adenocarcinoma. It is now recommended to perform routine foregut surveillance every 1 to 3 years once colonic polyposis is identified. This should be performed with a side-viewing upper endoscope to ensure direct viewing and biopsy of the ampulla and periampullary mucosa.

151. This is HNPCC. HNPCC is important—very important. You need to know about this condition. HNPCC is said to account for around 5% of all colorectal cancers, so for that reason alone it is vital to know all about this syndrome. Despite its prevalence, many internists and gastroenterologists remain poorly versed in the detection and appropriate surveillance of patients with HNPCC.

HNPCC is an autosomal dominant condition associated with a germline mutation in several different mismatch repair genes. The most prevalent mutations are MLH1 and MSH2. These mutations lead to microsatellite instability (MSI), which in turn promotes tumor progression. Patients with HNPCC do not have the same density of polyposis exhibited in FAP, but they do have a much higher overall risk of early polyposis compared to population controls. Colorectal cancer occurs in approximately 80% of affected patients. The median age of cancer formation is 46 years. Of note, the cancers in HNPCC tend to be right-sided, so flexible sigmoidoscopy is not adequate for surveillance, whereas flexible sigmoidoscopy is acceptable in FAP.

In addition to colon cancer, HNPCC is associated with a wide range of extracolonic malignancies. These include ureteral cancer (buzzword in this vignette), along with cancer of the ovaries, stomach, small intestine, and biliary tree. When these tumors are present, patients are classified as having the Muir-Torre variant of HNPCC. Diagnosing HNPCC has been somewhat controversial and can be confusing. The most commonly employed case-finding definition is based on the Amsterdam II criteria, which employs the so-called "3-2-1 rule." According to these criteria, HNPCC requires 3 or more close relatives (1 a first-degree relative of the other 2) spanning at least 2 generations, with at least 1 HNPCC-related cancer diagnosed before the age of 50. Whereas the Amsterdam I criteria are limited to colon cancer, Amsterdam II criteria are more liberal, and allow any HNPCC-related malignancy, including those listed above.

If a patient does not meet all the criteria, but HNPCC is still suspected, then further testing may confirm the diagnosis. In particular, if the patient has an affected family member with colon cancer, and if the cancer tissue is available, the tumor itself can be tested for MSI. If there is no tumor available, the patient can be tested with immunohistochemistry for MLH1 and MSH2. It gets more complicated than this.

For a full mind-blowing algorithm, refer to the American Gastroenterological Association guidelines on Hereditary Colorectal Cancer and Genetic Testing (*Gastroenterology* 2001;121:195-197). I have looked at that algorithm many times, and am personally unable to recall all the nuances and details without looking it up again. I would be surprised if that level of detail is tested on the Board exam. But, you should certainly know about MSI, MLH1, and MSH2 testing, in general.

152. This is tuberous sclerosis. Tuberous sclerosis is an autosomal dominant neurocutaneous disorder marked by abnormal cell cycle regulation. The condition presents with a striking range of abnormalities across nearly every organ system.

In the GI tract, patients with tuberous sclerosis develop diffuse hamartomas. They may also develop colonic ganglioneuromas, which are tumors composed of interlacing bundles of ganglion and Schwann cells. Extraintestinal manifestations of tuberous sclerosis are extensive, and include facial angiofibromas (buzzword in this vignette), which appear like little bumps in the nose and malar region of the face. Other features of tuberous sclerosis include mental retardation, epilepsy, bone cysts, cardiac rhabdomyoma, and renal cysts, among many other manifestations.

153. This is Turcot's Syndrome. Turcot's Syndrome is a subset of FAP in which patients have brain tumors. The most common brain tumors are medulloblastomas and gliomas.

154. This is Cowden's Syndrome. See Vignette 44 for details.

155. This is Peutz-Jegher's Syndrome (PJS). PJS is an autosomal dominant polyposis syndrome arising from a mutation in a gene on chromosome 9 that encodes a serine threonine kinase. It presents with diffuse hamartomatous polyps throughout the GI tract, along with characteristic hyperpigmentation on the lips and buccal mucosa. The hamartomas can become large and lead to GI bleeding, intussusception, recurrent abdominal pain, and bowel obstruction. Malignant transformation of hamartomatous polyps is rare, but it can occur. As the polyps get larger, the risk of malignant transformation increases. Patients with PJS also suffer from extraintestinal malignancies, including Sertoli cell testicular tumors in men (buzzword in this vignette) and ovarian sex-cord tumors in women.

Here's the Point!

Learn the (Painful) Table Below

Table 150-1
BUZZWORDS FOR HEREDITARY COLORECTAL CANCER SYNDROMES

Board Buzzword	Associated Condition(s)
Ampullary cancer	FAP
Angiofibromas	Tuberous Sclerosis
Bone cysts	Tuberous Sclerosis
Biliary tract malignancy	HNPCC (Muir-Torre Variant)
Cardiac rhabdomyomas	Tuberous Sclerosis
Congenital hypertrophy of the retinal pigmentation epithelium	Gardner's Syndrome
Desmoid tumors	Gardner's Syndrome
Duodenal cancer	FAP
Epidermoid cysts	Gardner's Syndrome
Epilepsy	Tuberous Sclerosis
Fibromas	Gardner's Syndrome
Ganglioneuromas	Tuberous Sclerosis
Gastric cancer	HNPCC (Muir-Torre Variant)
Gliomas	Turcot's Syndrome
Hamartomas	Peutz-Jegher's Syndrome; Cowden's Syndrome; Juvenile Polyposis; Tuberous Sclerosis
Hyperpigmentation of lips	Peutz-Jegher's Syndrome
Lipoma	Gardner's Syndrome
Medulloblastoma	Turcot's Syndrome
Mental retardation	Tuberous Sclerosis
Mesenteric fibromatosis	Gardner's Syndrome
Osteoma	Gardner's Syndrome
Ovarian cancer	HNPCC; Peutz-Jegher's Syndrome (sex-cord tumor)
Renal cysts	Tuberous Sclerosis
Sebaceous cysts	Gardner's Syndrome
Sertoli Cell testicular tumor	Peutz-Jegher's Syndrome
Small intestinal cancer	HNPCC (Muir-Torre Variant)
Supernumerary teeth	Gardner's Syndrome
Trichilemmomas	Cowden's Syndrome
Ureteral cancer	HNPCC (Muir-Torre Variant)

Vignettes 156-160: Villous Atrophy Run-Down

When you think of villous atrophy, you probably think of celiac sprue. That is good, because celiac sprue is incredibly prevalent (1 in 133 Americans). But there are many other conditions that cause villous atrophy. Below is a collection of patients found to have villous atrophy on jejunal biopsy. For each one, identify the underlying condition that caused the villous atrophy.

156. A 40-year-old man presents with chronic diarrhea. Small bowel biopsy reveals a plasma cell infiltrate, increased crypt depth, and evidence of shortened villi. There are trophozoites adherent to the enterocyte surface—they are not within the epithelium or subepithelium. The trophozoites have eyelike double nuclei and are flagellated.

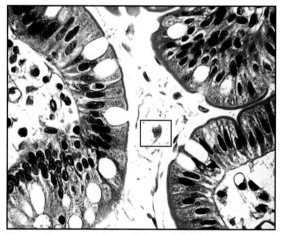

Figure 156-1. Small bowel biopsy. (Courtesy of Wilfred Weinstein, MD David Geffen School of Medicine at UCLA.)

157. A patient develops chronic diarrhea after visiting Haiti. He has a high MCV anemia and villous blunting on jejunal biopsy.

158. A 22-year-old woman with a history of hypothyroidism presents with chronic diarrhea. She has iron deficiency anemia, a low carotene, and villous atrophy on jejunal biopsy. Peripheral smear reveals Howell-Jolly bodies.

159. A 30-year-old man presents with chronic diarrhea and abdominal pain. He has a history of asthma and eczema. Jejunal biopsy reveals villous blunting along with a dense eosinophilic infiltrate exceeding 25 cells per high-power field.

160. A 50-year-old woman presents with diarrhea, abdominal pain, and acid reflux symptoms. Endoscopy reveals thick gastric folds, voluminous gastric secretions, and post bulbar duodenal ulcers. Jejunal biopsy reveals villous atrophy.

Vignettes 156-160: Answers

156. This is giardiasis. Although giardia does not invade the intestinal mucosa, it can nonetheless lead to mucosal blunting and frank atrophy in severe cases. Biopsy will reveal flagellated trophozoites with characteristic "eyelike" nuclei. A related condition is Chronic Variable Immunodeficiency (CVID). CVID may be associated with mucosal atrophy, and also presents with giardiasis. Unlike normal giardiasis, where there are underlying plasma cells, patients with CVID have trophozoites without a plasma cell infiltrate. See Vignette 139 for details.

157. This is tropical sprue. See Vignette 66 for details.

158. This is celiac sprue. I snuck this in despite the introductory comments that conditions other than celiac sprue cause villous blunting. Clues here include the younger age, history of hypothyroidism (Hashimoto's thyroiditis, in particular, is comorbid with celiac sprue), iron deficiency anemia, Howell-Jolly bodies (rare but well-described association with celiac sprue), and low carotene (indicating fat malabsorption).

159. This is eosinophilic enteritis. Patients with eosinophilic GI disorders often have comorbid atopic dermatitis, asthma, and eczema. When severe, eosinophilic enteritis can lead to villous blunting.

160. This is Zollinger Ellison Syndrome (ZES). The hyperchlorhydria of ZES can lead to damage of the duodenal and jejunal enterocytes. Both the villi and epithelial cells become inflamed, atrophic, and ultimately dysfunctional. In addition, patients with ZES have intraluminal inactivation of pancreatic enzymes. Thus, ZES leads to both malabsorption and maldigestion—the former from villous atrophy, the latter from enzyme activation. Diarrhea is common in ZES, as occurred here. The classic endoscopic appearance of ZES includes thick gastric folds, voluminous gastric juice, and multiple gastric, bulbar, and, most specifically, postbulbar ulcerations.

As an aside, there are other conditions that may present with villous blunting. These include Graft Versus Host Disease (GVHD), bacterial overgrowth, Crohn's Disease, intestinal lymphangiectasia (see Vignette 68), and cow's milk allergy, among others.

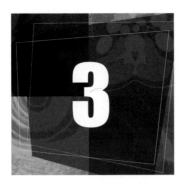

100 Board Review "Clinical Threshold Values"

There are many exam questions that require test takers to memorize some numerical threshold value, like: *"If the stool anion gap is less than XX, then it's secretory diarrhea."* Or: *"If a subepithelial gastric mass is larger than Y cm, it must come out."* These have been mentioned throughout the book. What follows is a "one-stop shop" for all these little numerical facts. These are presented by increasing numerical order—not by a rational taxonomy. So the resulting list will seem like a pretty random hodgepodge, which is the point. Exam questions are random too, so just go with the flow.

1 cm = If a gallbladder polyp gets bigger than this, then it should be removed regardless of symptoms, age, or presence of gallstones. Smaller lesions may still need to be removed, but not necessarily. See Vignette 28 for details.

1 cm = If a perigastric lymph node exceeds this size in the setting of a gastric GIST, then the risk of underlying malignancy of the GIST is high and resection is warranted. See Vignette 94 for details.

1.1 = If the serum ascites albumin gradient (SAAG) exceeds this value, then transudative processes are likely (eg, heart failure if total protein is above 2.5, cirrhosis if total protein is below 2.5). If it is below this value, then exudative processes are likely (eg, infection or malignancy).

1.5 = If the ALT:LDH ration exceeds this in the setting of severe transaminemia (eg, ALT and AST in 1,000+ range), then acute viral hepatitis is likely. If lower, consider drug-induced, toxin-induced, or hypoxemic-induced liver injury.

2 cm = If an appendiceal carcinoid exceeds this size, then a hemicolectomy is indicated. If it is smaller than this, then appendectomy is indicated (assuming no metastatic spread).

2 cm = If liver nodule exceeds 2 cm in a patient with cirrhosis, then it is considered hepatocellular cancer, assuming the lesion reveals evidence of hypervascularization on both triphasic CT and MRI with gadolinium. If the lesion exceeds 2 cm but is only hypervascular appearing on 1 of the 2 imaging techniques, then it is still considered hepatocellular cancer so long as the alfa fetoprotein also exceeds 400 ng/mL (another threshold). Confusing, but something you just need to memorize. See Table 120-1 for details.

2 cm = If an esophageal fibrovascular polyp exceeds this size, then surgery is indicated. If it is smaller, then snare polypectomy is warranted (assuming no significant penetrating vessels—see Vignette 4 for details).

2 cm = This is the minimum margin for rectal cancer resection. So tumors within 2 cm of the anal sphincter are generally not amenable to sphincter-preserving surgery and require an abdominoperineal resection (APR). Rectal tumors beyond 2 cm can often be treated with a sphincter-preserving surgery, such as a low anterior resection (LAR) or coloanal anastomosis.

2 cm = If a passed gallstone exceeds this size, then it will get stuck in the ileocecal valve and cause gallstone ileus (usually erodes directly from gallbladder into duodenum—too large to pass through biliary tract). See Vignette 81 for details.

2x ULN = If the ALP exceeds this upper limit of normal (ULN) threshold in the setting of a culprit medication (eg, erythromycin, estrogen, rifampin, amoxicillin, chlorpromazine), then drug-induced cholestasis is likely. Similarly, if the ALP/AST ratio exceeds 2, then this is a supportive criterion for canalicular ("bland") type cholestasis. See Vignette 69 for details.

2 weeks = Don't do a swallow evaluation until this much time has passed after a stroke. Premature swallow evaluation may be misleading, because swallowing function may return if you wait long enough. But 2 weeks is enough—if there is inadequate return of function by 2 weeks, it is unlikely to return rapidly thereafter (though may certainly return with time nonetheless).

2 minutes = If a patient cannot expel a 50- to 60-cc rectal balloon within this time frame, then the balloon expulsion test is consistent with pelvic dyssynergia. See Vignette 24 for details.

3 cm = If a gastrointestinal stromal tumor (GIST) in the 4th layer of the stomach exceeds this diameter, then surgery is indicated. If smaller, it all depends! See Vignette 94 for details.

3 cm = If an intraductal papillary mucinous tumor (IPMN) of the pancreas exceeds 3 cm, then a Whipple resection is warranted, regardless of other clinical features or parameters. See Vignette 111 for details.

3 cm = If a length of Barrett's mucosa is less, then it is considered "short segment Barrett's." However, this is now an outdated concept, as the risk of dysplasia is considered similar whether Barrett's is short segment or long segment.

3 cm = Maximum allowable size for multifocal hepatocellular cancer in order to still remain eligible for liver transplantation, assuming there are no more than 3 total nodules (Milan Criterion—see "5 cm" threshold, below, for additional Milan criterion).

pH of 4 = If intragastric pH rises above this threshold, then pepsin is inactivated and a pro-coagulant state is supported. This is the first goal of using a PPI in GI bleeding—to raise intragastric pH above 4, and preferably 6 (see threshold further below). Also, if intraesophageal pH falls below this threshold during pH-metry, it is considered an acid reflux event.

4 markers = When performing functional testing for constipation with radio-opaque markers (eg, Sitzmark study), the presence of more than 4 of the original 24 markers in the colon after 120 hours indicates slow transit constipation.

pH of 5 = In the setting of diarrhea with a high stool anion gap, if the stool pH is lower than this threshold, then think carbohydrate malabsorption. See Vignette 135 for details.

5 cm = If a hepatic adenoma exceeds this size, then it requires surgical excision. See Vignette 114 for details.

5 cm = Minimum margin for (non-rectal) colon cancer resection.

5 cm = Maximum allowable size for a solitary hepatocellular cancer in order to still remain eligible for liver transplantation (Milan Criterion).

5 crypts = If fewer than 5 crypts demonstrate high-grade dysplasia in Barrett's mucosa, and if there are no other foci of dysplasia identified, then the high-grade is considered "focal" high-grade dysplasia.

5x ULN = If the AST exceeds this threshold in autoimmune hepatitis (AIH), and the gamma globulin concurrently exceeds >2x the ULN, then initiate medical therapy. Of course, there are other indications to begin treatment for AIH.

5 mm = If esophageal mucosal breaks are smaller than 5 mm in erosive esophagitis, then it meets criteria for mild (Grade A) disease based on the Los Angeles Classification system. If larger, then it meets criteria for L.A. Class B.

5 cm = Usual position that pH catheter is placed above the lower esophageal sphincter during a 24-hour pH monitor.

5 mg/dL = BUN risk threshold to score a point for BUN elevation on 48-hour Ranson's criteria.

6 Liters = Fluid sequestration threshold to score a point for third spacing on 48-hour Ranson's criteria.

pH of 6 = When intragastric pH rises above this threshold, then platelet aggregation is enhanced. This is the second goal of using a PPI in GI bleeding—to raise intragastric pH above 4, first (see threshold above), and then above 6.

BD-IPMN

6 mm = If the pancreatic duct exceeds this diameter in the setting of a branch duct type intraductal papillary mucinous tumor (IPMN) of the pancreas, then a Whipple operation is warranted. See Vignette 111 for details.

6-7 mm = If the pancreatic duct exceeds this diameter in the setting of chronic pancreatitis, then a Peustow operation (ie, lateral pancreaticojejunostomy) can be considered. If smaller, then the success of this operation is low.

7.5 g = If more than this amount of 7.5 g acetaminophen is consumed at once, then acetaminophen can be hepatotoxic. Patients with an ingestion exceeding this threshold (or 150 mg/kg), and for whom a serum level is unavailable, should receive empiric N-acetyl-cysteine.

8 to 12 hours = When a disc battery is ingested and lodged in the esophagus, it can lead to esophageal perforation within 8 to 12 hours. Endoscopic removal must occur prior to this time period elapsing.

8 years = If pan-colitis has been present for this long in ulcerative colitis, then start colonoscopic surveillance for colorectal cancer (see "15 years" threshold, below, for a related threshold in ulcerative colitis).

8 mg/dL = Calcium threshold to score a point for calcium drop on 48-hour Ranson's criteria.

8 mm Hg = The lower esophageal sphincter pressure should fall below this in health. It typically exceeds this relaxation pressure in achalasia.

10% = If gastric retention of a test meal exceeds this threshold 4 hours into a scintigraphic emptying study, then the study is consistent with gastroparesis.

10% = If the local *H. pylori* prevalence exceeds this threshold, then *H. pylori* "test-and-treat" is the first line approach in uninvestigated dyspepsia. If below this threshold, then empiric PPI therapy is warranted.

10% = Hematocrit threshold to score a point for Hct drop on 48-hour Ranson's criteria.

10x ULN = If the AST exceeds this threshold in AIH, then initiate medical therapy regardless of the gamma globulin level.

10 mmol/L = The goal of diuretic therapy is to induce natriuresis, defined by a spot urine sodium exceeding this threshold.

10 cm = If an echinoccal liver cyst exceeds this size, then it likely requires surgery for definitive therapy due to high risk of rupture.

10 to 12 cm = If the cecum diameter exceeds this threshold in Ogilvie's syndrome, then the risk of perforation increases significantly. Neostigmine is warranted in this setting (see Vignette 80 for details).

10 to 30 mm Hg = Normal resting tone of LES.

10 mm Hg = Target pressure less than this for LES in achalasia after dilation.

12 mm = Critical narrowing for esophageal dysphagia onset.

12 hours = Need to get out impacted food by this time in order to minimize esophageal pressure necrosis.

12 mm = In type I sphincter of Oddi dysfunction, if the common bile duct exceeds this size, then sphincterotomy is indicated.

12 mm Hg = If the hepatic venous pressure gradient (HVPG) exceeds this, then variceal formation is enhanced. Goal of beta blocker therapy is to reduce beneath this threshold.

15 years = Consider periodic endoscopic surveillance after having a diagnosis of achalasia for this period of time.

15 cm = Average distance from incisors to upper esophageal sphincter (ie, crycopharyngeus).

15 yrs = If left-sided colitis has been present for this period of time, then begin colorectal cancer surveillance in ulcerative colitis.

15 to 25 per high power field = Eosinophilic esophagitis is diagnosed when the density of eosinophils per high power field on microscopy of esophageal biopsies exceeds this threshold.

15 to 30 grams = Target daily intake of dietary fiber for patients with chronic constipation.

20 mm Hg = Goal of treatment in acute liver failure complicated by intracranial pressure (ICP) is to drop intracranial pressure below this threshold.

20 mg/dL = Ceruloplasmin levels below this are sensitive (but not specific) for Wilson disease.

20 cm = Average distance from incisors to aortic arch.

20% = If non-propagating high pressure waves occur in at least 20% of wet swallows during manometry, then criteria are met for diffuse esophageal spasm (DES). See Vignette 104 for details.

20-100 polyps = If more than 20 adenomatous polyps identified (but less than 100), then may be attenuated form of familial adenomatous polyposis (FAP).

25 cm = Average distance from incisors to main-stem bronchus.

25 = Lymphocytic gastritis is diagnosed when the density of lymphocytes per high power field on microscopy of gastric biopsies exceeds this threshold.

30 mm Hg = If simultaneous esophageal pressure waves exceed this pressure in at least 20% of wet swallows on manometry, then criteria are met for diffuse esophageal spasm. See Vignette 104 for details.

32 = If Maddrey's Discriminant Function Score (4.6 x ΔPT + total bilirubin) is above this in alcoholic hepatitis, then start steroids or pentoxiphylline.

35 = If BMI is higher and there are comorbid complications of obesity, then bariatric surgery is appropriate.

36 hours = Average normal colonic transit time.

40 = If BMI is higher, then bariatric surgery is appropriate regardless of comorbid complications.

40 cm = Average distance from incisors to gastroesophageal junction.

40 mm Hg = The lower esophageal sphincter pressure exceeds this threshold in achalasia.

50 =   If CD4 count falls below 50, then MAC risk increases. So, if bloody diarrhea with CD4 below 50, think about MAC colitis in the differential diagnosis.

50 =   Goal in hereditary hemochromatosis is to drive ferritin below this level.

50 =   If the stool anion gap (290-2[Na+K]) is lower in diarrhea, then the mechanism is most likely secretory diarrhea. See Vignette 135 for details.

50% = If the GERD symptom index—percentage of symptom events that occur during a documented acid reflux event (pH<4)—rises higher, then the index is considered clinically significant.

50 mm Hg = Goal is to keep cerebral pressure below this value in hepatic encephalopathy.

50 years = If a patient with reflux symptoms is older than this, then endoscopy is warranted regardless of presence vs absence of alarm signs and symptoms. See Vignettes 121-126 for details.

55 years = If a patient with nonreflux dyspepsia symptoms is older than this, then endoscopy is warranted regardless of presence vs absence of alarm signs and symptoms. See Vignettes 121-126 for details.

55 years = Age threshold to score a point for advanced age on admission Ranson's criteria.

60 cm = If more of terminal ileum is removed, then B12 deficiency results.

60 mm Hg = PaO2 threshold to score a point for oxygenation drop on 48 hour Ranson's criteria.

88 =   If platelet count below this in cirrhosis, then risk of underlying varices increases substantially.

90 minutes = During a hydrogen breath test for small intestinal bacterial overgrowth, any measurable peak prior to this time indicates a positive test (there are other methods as well, by the way—see other thresholds). See Vignette 134 for details.

100 = If more colonic adenomatous polyps, then may be FAP.

100 cm = If more of the terminal ileum is removed, then patient may deplete bile acid pool and develop diarrhea from fat malabsorption. Treatment with medium chain triglycerides is warranted. See Vignette 130 for details.

100 mcg/ 24 hours = Urinary copper excretion above this is found in most all symptomatic Wilson disease patients.

100 days = Divides acute versus chronic graft vs host disease (GVHD).

180 =   If the CD4 count falls below this, then cryptosporidium risk increases. So, if watery diarrhea with CD4 below this level, think about cryptosporidiosis in the differential diagnosis. See Vignette 7 for details.

180 mm Hg = Peak esophageal pressure must exceed this in order to meet criteria for nutcracker esophagus. See Vignette 104 for details.

180 minutes = During a hydrogen breath test for small intestinal bacterial overgrowth, a >20 part per million rise prior to this time indicates a positive test (there are other methods as well, by the way—see other thresholds). See Vignette 134 for details.

192 = If the CEA level is above this in a pancreatic cyst, then it is concerning for malignancy. See Vignette 111 for details.

200 = If the serum gastrin increases by more than this in a patient with hypergastrinemia after receiving an injection of secretin, then the secretin stimulation test is positive and Zollinger Ellison Syndrome is likely. See Vignettes 29-33 for details.

200 mg/dL = Glucose threshold to score a point for glucose elevation on admission Ranson's criteria.

235 = The therapeutic goal with azathirprine/6-MP is to keep 6-thioguanine (6-TG) levels above this threshold. Lower levels yield poor efficacy.

250 = If the PMN count in ascites exceeds this value in cirrhosis, then the patient has spontaneous bacterial peritonitis (SBP). See Vignettes 17-22 for details.

250 U/L = AST threshold to score a point for AST elevation on admission Ranson's criteria.

350 IU/L = LDH threshold to score a point for LDH elevation on admission Ranson's criteria.

450 = 6-TG levels above this can be myelotoxic when using azathioprine/6-MP.

1000 = If gastrin higher, then consider Zollinger Ellison Syndrome. See Vignettes 29-33 for details.

5700 = 6-MMP levels above this may be hepatotoxic when using azathioprine/6-MP.

16,000/mm^3 = White blood cell threshold to score a point for WBC elevation on admission Ranson's criteria.

10^5 colony forming units = If higher bacterial count measure in a jejunal aspirate, then there is small intestinal bacterial overgrowth. See Vignette 134 for details.

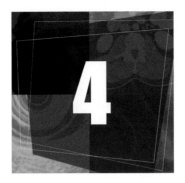

"CRUNCH-TIME" SELF TEST—
TIME TO GET YOUR GAME ON

This is a rapid-fire "crunch-time" self test. The questions in this test are loosely based on the "here's the point" bullet points from each of the vignettes. These represent the distilled essence of potential Board vignettes, so know them well. As you read each one-liner, write in the diagnosis in the corresponding blank line. Really... just actively write it in, right there on the page. Although Board questions often ask about much more than the mere diagnosis, you will need to know the diagnosis first in order to know what to do next. So this is a bottom-line test of your basic diagnostic capabilities for the "tough stuff" that might show up on the exam.

Few of these are true "gimmies." If you've carefully studied the vignettes up to this point, then this should be a relative snap—and should reaffirm that you are well on your way to acing the tough stuff. Some of these are stand-alone questions that do not have a corresponding vignette in the book.

Once you have finished the test, which may take a few sessions depending on how much time you are allotting for this activity, check with the answer key on page 225 and score yourself according to the interpretation guide on page 233. Try not to cheat too much—just write down your best guess prior to checking the answer, and then add up all the correct answers you get once you're done (no partial credit).

If you cheat your way through this (like I always do when I'm stuck on a crossword puzzle), then you won't really know how you did and won't be able to interpret your score according to the guide on page 233. If you are in crunch time, then once you are through scoring yur test, be sure to look up the corresponding vignettes for each of the items you got wrong, and then study those vignettes carefully to fill in your knowledge gaps.

Question 1. Hamartomatous polyps in the colon and coalescing mucosal lesions in the buccal mucosa with "cobblestoning" of the tongue (yep, started with a hard one—don't cheat yet!)

▶ Diagnosis_____

Question 2. Cyanosis with normal oxygen saturation after using Hurricane Spray before endoscopy.

▶ Diagnosis_____

✻**Question 3.** Fever, weight loss, costovertebral angle tenderness, microscopic hematuria, and isolated elevated ALP level with normal transaminases.

▶ Diagnosis_____

Question 4. Heart fibrosis and right heart failure with elevated chromogranin A.

▶ Diagnosis_____

Question 5. Pathergic skin lesion on lower extremity in a patient with ulcerative colitis.

▶ Diagnosis_____

Question 6. Diarrhea + Cruise Ship.

▶ Diagnosis_____

Question 7. Necrolytic migratory erythema.

▶ Diagnosis_____

Question 8. 73-year-old with bony pain, weight loss, narrow anion gap, hypercalcemia, now presenting with upper GI hemorrhage and found to have gastric mass.

▶ Diagnosis_____

Question 9. Diarrhea + tropics + high MCV anemia.

▶ Diagnosis_____

Question 10. "Plucked chicken skin" + GI bleeding.

▶ Diagnosis_____

Question 11. Abdominal pain out of proportion to palpation with explosive maroon stools.

▶ Diagnosis_____

Question 12. Dysphagia + cervical "shelf" on upper GI series.

▶ Diagnosis_____

Question 13. Subepithelial gastric mass staining positive for CD117 (c-kit).

▶ Diagnosis_____

Question 14. Sitophobia from meal-related dyspepsia + Weight Loss + Epigastric Bruit + Concave indentation on celiac trunk on angiography.

▶ Diagnosis_____

Question 15. Crohn's disease with sharp CVA tenderness and hematuria.

▶ Diagnosis_____

Question 16. Pancreatic cyst on CT with mucinous, gelatinous fluid from ampulla on endoscopy.

▶ Diagnosis_____

Question 17. Diarrhea + PAS-positive foamy macrophages on small intestinal biopsy + <u>negative</u> acid fast stain.

▶ Diagnosis_____

Question 18. Diarrhea + PAS-positive foamy macrophages on small intestinal biopsy + <u>positive</u> acid fast stain.

▶ Diagnosis_____

Question 19. HIV Diarrhea + Paresthsia in "saddle distribution."

▶ Diagnosis_____

Question 20. HIV + Bloody Diarrhea + "Flask-Like Ulcers" on biopsy.

▶ Diagnosis_____

Question 21. HIV + Bloody Diarrhea + "Owl's Eyes" inclusions on biopsy.

▶ Diagnosis_____

Question 22. Recurrent tongue swelling + fissured tongue + facial paralysis + noncaseating granulomas of tongue + diarrhea.

▶ Diagnosis_____

Question 23. Subepithelial gastric mass + 4th layer involvement + actin-positive + CD 117-negative.

▶ Diagnosis_____

Question 24. Acute lower abdominal pain in the setting of a focal oval area of fat in anti-mesenteric border of the sigmoid colon on CT with a central attenuating line through the inflamed fat.

▶ Diagnosis_____

Question 25. Diarrhea + "congophilic angiopathy."

▶ Diagnosis_____

Question 26. Diarrhea + high MCV + low B12 level + high folate level.

▸ Diagnosis_____

Question 27. Dyspepsia + thick gastric folds + foveolar hyperplasia.

▸ Diagnosis_____

Question 28. High transferrin saturation + Kupffer cells infiltrated with iron + hepatocytes not infiltrated.

▸ Diagnosis_____

Question 29. Isolated fundic varices in setting of chronic pancreatitis.

▸ Diagnosis_____

Question 30. Ascites + elevated bilirubin + hepatomegaly + bone marrow transplant within previous 3 weeks.

▸ Diagnosis_____

Question 31. Constipation with simultaneous increase in both rectal and anal leads on anorectal manometry.

▸ Diagnosis_____

Question 32. Hamartomatous polyps + protein-losing enteropathy + diarrhea + alopecia + dystrophic nails.

▸ Diagnosis_____

Question 33. Weird Oral Projection + Globus + Dysphagia.

▸ Diagnosis_____

Question 34. Gastric polyps with cystic dilatations of oxyntic gland mucosa in setting of PPI use.

▸ Diagnosis_____

Question 35. PAS-positive, diastase-resistant globules accumulated in hepatocytes.

▸ Diagnosis_____

Question 36. Young woman with diarrhea, iron deficiency anemia, and low carotene.

▸ Diagnosis_____

Question 37. High serum calcium + thick gastric folds + multiple gastric ulcers.

▸ Diagnosis_____

Question 38. Recurrent biliary colic + elevated amylase + high AST during symptoms + dilated common bile duct + no stones on ultrasound.

▸ Diagnosis_____

Question 39. Most likely diagnosis in a pregnant woman who turned yellow (yeah, that's all you get).

▸ Diagnosis_____

Question 40. Vasculopath + Anemia + "Needle shaped clefts" on mucosal biopsies of colon.

▸ Diagnosis_____

Question 41. Hematemesis + Subcutaneous Air + Left-Sided Effusion.

▸ Diagnosis_____

Question 42. Elevated gastrin + low intragastric pH + hypertrophic parietal cell mass + negative secretin stimulation test.

▶ Diagnosis_____

Question 43. Alopecia + Dystrophic Nails + Colon Polyps.

▶ Diagnosis_____

Question 44. HIV + Fever + Diarrhea + B12 Deficiency.

▶ Diagnosis_____

Question 45. Thick Gastric Folds + Diarrhea + Low Albumin + Protein Losing Enteropathy + Edema.

▶ Diagnosis_____

Question 46. Black Velvety Rash + No Metabolic Syndrome + Early Satiety + Dyspepsia + Weight Loss.

▶ Diagnosis_____

Question 47. Ascites with a PMN count <250 but positive for *E. coli*.

▶ Diagnosis_____

Question 48. Recurrent Abdominal Pain + Family History of Abdominal Syndrome + Visceral and Peripheral Edema + Worsens with Enalapril.

▶ Diagnosis_____

Question 49. Keratoderma of Palms and Soles + Dysphagia.

▶ Diagnosis_____

Question 50. AIDS + Jaundice + Cystic Blood-Filled Space on Liver Biopsy.

▶ Diagnosis_____

Question 51. Dyspepsia + Sheets of T Lymphocytes on Gastric Biopsies.

▶ Diagnosis_____

Question 52. Biggest concern in a patient with high-volume lower GI bleeding in the setting of a previous abdominal aortic aneurysm repair.

▶ Diagnosis_____

Question 53. Biggest concern in a patient developing high-volume lower GI bleeding within hours of a diagnostic liver biopsy.

▶ Diagnosis_____

Question 54. Female + Monthly Abdominal Cramping + Colonic Subepithelial Nodule During Flares + No Nodule Between Flares.

▶ Diagnosis_____

Question 55. Neutropenia + Right Lower Quadrant Abdominal Pain + Thickened Cecum on CT.

▶ Diagnosis_____

Question 56. Intermittent Vague Abdominal Pain + Bulbous Dilation of Ampulla on ERCP.

▶ Diagnosis_____

Question 57. Diarrhea + Erythematous Scaling Plaques on Legs and Face + Receiving TPN.

▶ Diagnosis_____

Question 58. Portal Hypertension + Eosinophilia + Normal Liver Function Tests + Large Spleen.

▶ Diagnosis_____

Question 59. Recurrent small bowel obstructions in the setting of hypercalcemia.

▶ Diagnosis_____

Question 60. Recalcitrant acid reflux symptoms post-Billroth II with markedly elevated gastrin levels.

▶ Diagnosis_____

Question 61. Cavernous Hemangioma on Mouth and Tongue + GI Bleeding + History of Intussusception.

▶ Diagnosis_____

Question 62. History of Chronic Pancreatitis + GI Bleed + Blood from Ampulla on Endoscopy.

▶ Diagnosis_____

Question 63. Isolated Elevated ALP + Bad Headaches + Markedly Elevated ESR.

▶ Diagnosis_____

Question 64. 36-year-old woman with chronic cough, bilateral hilar adenopathy, erythema nodosum and pancreatic head mass with dilated common bile duct in the setting of fevers and fatigue.

▶ Diagnosis_____

Question 65. Diarrhea + Chocolate Milk.

▶ Diagnosis_____

Question 66. Diarrhea + Reheated Rice.

▶ Diagnosis_____

Question 67. Diarrhea + Undercooked Beef.

▶ Diagnosis_____

Question 68. Diarrhea + Raw Shellfish from Gulf Coast.

▶ Diagnosis_____

Question 69. Patient on 6-MP for Crohn's Disease has leukopenia, markedly elevated 6-TG level, and low 6-MMP level.

▶ Diagnosis_____

Question 70. Diarrhea + Stool Anion Gap=130 + Stool pH>5.

▶ Diagnosis_____

Question 71. Subepithelial Gastric Nodule + Actin and Vimentin-Positive Staining.

▶ Diagnosis_____

Question 72. Subepithelial Gastric Nodule + S100-positive Staining.

▶ Diagnosis_____

Question 73. Subepithelial gastric nodule that is spherical, extramural and anechoic on endoscopic ultrasound.

▶ Diagnosis_____

Question 74. Yellow + Panniculitis + History of Arterial Dissection.

▶ Diagnosis_____

Question 75. Smoker + New-onset achalasia + Anti-Hu antibody.

▶ Diagnosis_____

Question 76. Recurrent giardiasis with virtually no plasma cells on mucosal biopsies of the proximal jejunum.

▶ Diagnosis_____

Question 77. Interface hepatitis with a plasma cell infiltrate.

▶ Diagnosis_____

Question 78. Diarrhea + ≥100cm of Terminal Ileum removed.

▶ Diagnosis_____

Question 79. Jaundice and mental status changes at week 38 of pregnancy with elevated bilirubin, elevated INR, and low serum glucose.

▶ Diagnosis_____

Question 80. Abdominal pain and left pleural effusion 3 weeks after motor vehicle accident.

▶ Diagnosis_____

Question 81. Tumor from a 38-year-old with colon cancer is found to have microsatellite instability and to express MLH1 and MSH2. There is an extensive family history of colon cancer.

▶ Diagnosis_____

Question 82. Dysphagia + "Megaduodenum" on barium study.

▶ Diagnosis_____

Question 83. Dysphagia + Living Under a "Thatched Roof Hut."

▶ Diagnosis_____

Question 84. Recurrent Pancreatitis + Elevated IgG-4.

▸ Diagnosis_____

Question 85. Abdominal Pain + Positive "Carnett Sign."

▸ Diagnosis_____

Question 86. Angular Stomatitis + Glossitis + Seborrheic Dermatitis + Visual Changes + Cheilosis.

▸ Diagnosis_____

Question 87. Diarrhea + Dermatitis + Dementia.

▸ Diagnosis_____

Question 88. TPN + Night Blindness + Tachycardia + Vomiting + Recurrent Headaches + Shortness of Breath.

▸ Diagnosis_____

Question 89. Young patient from Mediterranean region with a recent *Campylobacter* infection who now has a dense lyphoplasmacytic inflitrate in the small intestine and a heavy chain paraproteinemia.

▸ Diagnosis_____

Question 90. TPN + Heart Failure + Myositis.

▸ Diagnosis_____

Question 91. Chronic Diarrhea + Pruritic Rash on Extensor Surfaces of Arms.

▸ Diagnosis_____

Question 92. Young male from Turkey with intermittent bouts of overwhelming abdominal pain, elevated ESR, and a family history of the same.

▸ Diagnosis_____

Question 93. Severe Bloody Diarrhea + Discreet Ulcers in Colon + Ingested Erythrocytes in Motile Trophozoites on mucosal biopsy.

▸ Diagnosis_____

Question 94. Large volume watery diarrhea + Hypokalemia + Achlorhydria + Pancreatic mass.

▸ Diagnosis_____

Question 95. Recurrent abdominal pain + Blistering of hands + Neuropsychiatric history.

▸ Diagnosis_____

Question 96. Positive Rheumatoid Factor + Lower Extremity Purpuric Rash + Paresthesias + Hepatitis C.

▸ Diagnosis_____

Question 97. Small Bowel Obstruction + "Café au lait" Macules + Axillary Freckles.

▸ Diagnosis_____

Question 98. A 30-year-old with chronic recalcitrant constipation and intermittent fecal impaction fails a balloon expulsion test and, on barium enema, has a normal-sized rectum but severely dilated sigmoid colon.

▸ Diagnosis_____

Question 99. Acute Bloody Diarrhea + Fever + Thrombocytopenia + Renal Insufficiency + Rash.

▸ Diagnosis_____

Question 100. Angioid Streaks in Eyes + Isolated Elevated ALP.

▶ Diagnosis_____

Question 101. Fulminant Liver Failure + Markedly Depressed ALP.

▶ Diagnosis_____

Question 102. Health freak + Elevated liver tests + Lipid-filled stellate cells on liver biopsy.

▶ Diagnosis_____

Question 103. Flushing with alcohol ingestion + Intermittent hypotension + Darier's Sign + Abdominal pain + Malabsorption + Hepatosplenomegaly + Elevated ALP (this has to be something!)

▶ Diagnosis_____

Question 104. Critically ill patient + Fever + Elevated amylase + Thick gallbladder wall on ultrasound but no stones + Positive Murphy's sign.

▶ Diagnosis_____

Question 105. Teenager with recurrent abdominal pain in the setting of chronic renal insufficiency, arthralgias, and intermittent rash over buttocks and lower extremities.

▶ Diagnosis_____

Question 106. Teenager with recurrent abdominal pain, diarrhea, and colitis in the setting of asthma.

▶ Diagnosis_____

Question 107. Diabetes + Gallstones + Weight loss + Steatorrhea + Pancreatic mass.

▶ Diagnosis_____

Question 108. Torrential upper GI hemorrhage in setting of enlarged atria and quinidine use.

▶ Diagnosis_____

Question 109. Dysphagia + Right subclavian artery aberrantly arising from left aortic arch.

▶ Diagnosis_____

Question 110. Vitiligo+ Hypergastrinemia.

▶ Diagnosis_____

Question 111. Weight loss + "Double duct sign" on ERCP.

▶ Diagnosis_____

Question 112. History of gallstones + Recurrent cholecystitis + Small bowel obstruction at ileocecal valve.

▶ Diagnosis_____

Question 113. Young woman + Liver mass with central stellate scar on CT.

▶ Diagnosis_____

Question 114. Diabetes + Dermatitis + Diarrhea + Weight loss + Pancreatic Mass.

▶ Diagnosis_____

Question 115. Elderly patient with asymptomatic pearly white papules throughout the esophagus that are negative for hyphal forms.

▶ Diagnosis_____

Question 116. ICU patient with obstipation and abdominal distension, CT reveals no evidence of obstruction but demonstrates a cecal diameter >10cm.

▸ Diagnosis_____

Question 117. Pancreatic cysts + Retinal angiomatosis + CNS hemangioblastoma.

▸ Diagnosis_____

Question 118. Hepatitis C + Purple, polygonal, pruritic papules on lower extremities.

▸ Diagnosis_____

Question 119. Patient with cirrhosis develops blistering skin lesions and septic shock after eating seafood.

▸ Diagnosis_____

Question 120. Sudden onset of seborrheic keratoses in elderly patients with recent unintended weight loss.

▸ Diagnosis_____

Question 121. AIDS patient on PPIs for dyspepsia has recalcitrant esophageal candidiasis despite two courses of fluconazole.

▸ Diagnosis_____

Question 122. Teenager with lifelong diarrhea + Contraction alkalosis + High chloride concentration in stool.

▸ Diagnosis_____

Question 123. Young man with recurrent bouts of vomiting for years and migraine headaches in the setting of marijuana use.

▸ Diagnosis_____

Question 124. Teenager with recurrent abdominal pain, jaundice, and an abdominal mass, with an ERCP revealing a cystic dilatation of the intraduodenal portion of the common bile duct.

▸ Diagnosis_____

Question 125. Diarrhea + Pet turtle.

▸ Diagnosis_____

Question 126. "Stepwise" fever + Abdominal pain + Temperature-pulse dissociation + "Rose spots" on trunk and abdomen.

▸ Diagnosis_____

Question 127. HBsAg(+), HBsAb(-), HBeAg(-), HBeAb(+), HBV DNA>10^5.

▸ Diagnosis_____

Question 128. Most likely diagnosis in patient with AIDS, CD4<200, with discreet elongated mid-esophageal ulcer that is negative for HSV, CMV, and Candida on brushings and biopsy.

▸ Diagnosis_____

Question 129. Patient with celiac sprue has persistent diarrhea despite compliance with diet and reversal of small bowel Marsh lesions.

▸ Diagnosis_____

Question 130. Diarrhea after terminal ileal surgery with <100 cm removed.

▸ Diagnosis_____

Question 131. Polyposis + "3-2-1 Rule" positive in family.

▸ Diagnosis_____

Question 132. Asian immigrant + Recurrent pyogenic cholangitis + Intra- and extrahepatic stone disease + Diffuse bile duct dilatations and strictures.

▶ Diagnosis_____

Question 133. Elevated transaminases + Arthritis in 2nd and 3rd MCP joints.

▶ Diagnosis_____

Question 134. Swimming in Lake + Elevated ALP/TB + Temperature-pulse dissociation.

▶ Diagnosis_____

Question 135. Recurrent bloody diarrhea after ileostomy that improves with short chain fatty acid enemas.

▶ Diagnosis_____

Question 136. Young patient + Ataxia + Chronic diarrhea + Low serum carotene + Lipid-containing vacuoles in enterocytes on small bowel biopsy.

▶ Diagnosis_____

Question 137. Severe pruritis at week 30 of pregnancy with elevated serum bile acid levels.

▶ Diagnosis_____

Question 138. Patient with Crohn's Disease has hard, painful, inflamed lumps with pus drainage under armpit.

▶ Diagnosis_____

Question 139. Patient with chronic obstructive pulmonary disease is found to have a submucosal rounded mass in the sigmoid colon during screening colonoscopy. The mass is biopsied and subsequently "deflates" and nearly disappears.

▶ Diagnosis_____

Question 140. Steatorrhea + Gastroparesis + Enlarged Heart + Perhipheral Neuropathy + Liver Test Abnormalities.

▸ Diagnosis_____

Question 141. Patients with long-standing early satiety and nausea but no weight loss. Endoscopy reveals extrinsic compression of second part of duodenum. CT reveals enlarged head of the pancreas without a focal mass.

▸ Diagnosis_____

Question 142. Dysphagia + Erythematous Scaling Lesions on Knuckles + "Shawl Sign" on Nape of Neck.

▸ Diagnosis_____

Question 143. Patient is admitted for pancreatitis. You give Compazine (procholperazime) for recurrent nausea and vomiting. Within 30 minutes, the patient develops a high fever, altered mental status, and becomes stiff as a board.

▸ Diagnosis_____

Question 144. Paroxysmal and terrible anorectal pain that lasts seconds, and then is gone. Rectal exam and colonoscopy are normal.

▸ Diagnosis_____

Question 145. Nausea + Vomiting + Kidney Stones + Constipation + Muscle Aches + Weakness + Depression.

▸ Diagnosis_____

Question 146. Intermittent epigastric pain always accompanied by shortness of breath and diaphoresis. Epigastric pain usually triggered by exertion.

▸ Diagnosis_____

Question 147. Elevated ALP/GGT + Normal AST/ALT + Normal bilirubin + Morning stiffness in hands + Subcutaneous nodules along forearms.

▶ Diagnosis_____

Question 148. Colon Polyps + Epidermoid Cysts + Supernumerary Teeth + Osteoma.

▶ Diagnosis_____

Question 149. Premature graying + vitiligo + positive Rhomberg sign + elevated gastrin.

▶ Diagnosis_____

Question 150. Rheumatoid arthritis + splenomegaly + neutropenia + nodular regenerative hyperplasia + portal hypertension.

▶ Diagnosis_____

Question 151. Recent constipation + *Strep bovis* endocarditis.

▶ Diagnosis_____

Question 152. Patient with bloody diarrhea receives empiric antibiotics for presumed infectious colitis. The platelet count and hemoglobin subsequently fall and the creatinine rises. The patient has altered mental status and progressive fever.

▶ Diagnosis_____

Question 153. Low serum protein + Diarrhea + Focal white spots throughout small bowel mucosa.

▶ Diagnosis_____

Question 154. Alcoholic + Ataxia + Tachycardia + Acidosis.

▶ Diagnosis_____

Question 155. Diarrhea + Dysmotility + Heart Failure + Orthostatic Hypotension.

▶ Diagnosis_____

Question 156. HIV + Diarrhea + Eosinophilia + Developing Country + Charcot Leyden crystals in stool.

▶ Diagnosis_____

Question 157. Superficial Migratory Thrombophlebitis + Depression + Abdominal Pain.

▶ Diagnosis_____

Question 158. Recurrent Abdominal Pain + Recurrent Blistering on Dorsa of Hands + Hypertrichosis.

▶ Diagnosis_____

Question 159. Iron Deficiency Anemia + Esophageal Web.

▶ Diagnosis_____

Question 160. ↑Na +↓K +↓Cl +↑HC03 +↑BUN + Recurrent Vomiting.

▶ Diagnosis_____

Question 161. Pharyngeal dysphagia in an elderly patient with osteoarthritis and a history of repetitive traumatic neck injuries.

▶ Diagnosis_____

Question 162. Dysphagia + History of Eczema + "Rings" in Esophagus on Endoscopy.

▶ Diagnosis_____

Question 163. Woman on oral contraceptives has subcapsular hepatic mass on CT.

▸ Diagnosis_____

Question 164. Essential thrombocytosis + Elevated ALP / GGT + Multiple hypodense nodules in liver on CT.

▸ Diagnosis_____

Question 165. Chronic diarrhea with stool anion gap >100 and stool pH<5.

▸ Diagnosis_____

Question 166. Cholestasis + "Florid Duct Lesion" with Granulomas + Ductopenia.

▸ Diagnosis_____

Question 167. A 22-year-old with recurrent abdominal pain undergoes upper endoscopy which reveals focal patches of erythema. Biopsies are negative for *H. pylori*. His ESR and CRP are elevated.

▸ Diagnosis_____

Question 168. Technically challenging colonoscopy + Focal white patches with clear spaces on biopsy.

▸ Diagnosis_____

Question 169. Apthous ulcers in mouth and terminal ileum + Genital ulcer.

▸ Diagnosis_____

Question 170. Joint hypermobility + Splanchnic Aneurysms + Recurrent abdominal pain.

▸ Diagnosis_____

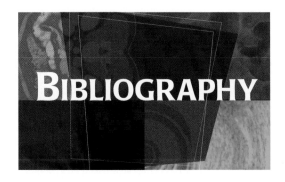

BIBLIOGRAPHY

Aberra FN. Infections of the biliary system. In: Ginsberg GG, Ahmad NA, eds. *The Clinician's Guide to Pancreaticobiliary Disorders*. Thorofare, NJ: SLACK Incorporated; 2006:121-146.

Abubakar I, Aliyu SH, Arumugam C, Hunter PR, Usman NK. Prevention and treatment of cryptosporidiosis in immunocompromised patients. *Cochrane Database Syst Rev.* 2007;24(1):CD004932.

Andrade RJ, Salmeron J, Lucena MI. Drug hepatotoxicity In: Reddy K, Faust T, editors. *The Clinician's Guide to Liver Disease*. Thorofare, NJ: SLACK Incorporated; 2006:321-343.

Bharucha AE, Wald A, Enck P, Rao S. Functional anorectal disorders.*Gastroenterology.* 2006;130:1510-1518.

Bjerke HS. Boerhaave's syndrome and barogenic injuries of the esophagus. *Chest Surg Clin N Am.* 1994;4(4):819-825.

Brandt LJ, Boley SJ. AGA technical review on intestinal ischemia. American Gastrointestinal Association. *Gastroenterology.* 2000;118(5):954-968.

Callahan RD, Reddy K. Liver disease in pregnancy. In: Reddy K, Faust T, editors. *The Clinician's Guide to Liver Disease*. Thorofare, NJ: SLACK Incorporated; 2006:211-230.

Coffey RJ, Washington MK, Corless CL, Heinrich MC. Ménétrier disease and gastrointestinal stromal tumors: hyper-proliferative disorders of the stomach. *J Clin Invest.* 2007;117(1):70-80.

Costanza CD, Longstreth GF, Liu AL. Chronic abdominal wall pain: clinical features, health care costs, and long-term outcome. *Clin Gastroenterol Hepatol.* 2004;2(5):395-399.

Davila ML. Neutropenic enterocolitis. *Curr Opin Gastroenterol.* 2006;22(1):44-47.

Domsic R, Fasanella K, Bielefeldt K. Gastrointestinal manifestations of systemic sclerosis. *Dig Dis Sci.* 2008;53(5):1163-1174.

Dore MP, Fattovich G, Sepulveda AR, Realidi G. Cryoglobulinemia related to hepatitis C virus infection. *Dig Dis Sci.* 2007;52(4):897-907.

Dubinsky MC, Lamothe S, Yang HY, et al. Pharmacogenomics and metabolite measurement for 6-mercaptopurine therapy in inflammatory bowel disease. *Gastroenterology.* 2000;118(4):705-713.

DuPont HL. Guidelines on acute infectious diarrhea in adults: the Practice Parameters Committee of the American College of Gastroenterology. *Am J Gastroenterol.* 1997;92(11):1962-1975.

Emory TS, Carpenter HA, Gostout CJ, Sobin LH, eds. *Atlas of Gastrointestinal Endoscopy & Endoscopic Biopsies*. Washington DC: Armed Forces Institute of Pathology (AFIP) Press; 2000.

Fine KD, Schiller LR. AGA technical review on the evaluation and management of chronic diarrhea. *Gastroenterology.* 1999;116(6):1464-1486.

Fine KD, Stone MJ. Alpha-heavy chain disease, Mediterranean lymphoma, and immunoproliferative small intestinal disease: a review of clinicopathological features, pathogenesis, and differential diagnosis. *Am J Gastroenterol.* 1999;94(5):1139-1152.

Fenollar F, Puechal X, Raoult D. Whipple's disease. *N Engl J Med.* 2007;356(1):55-66.

Gaya DR. Foulis AK, Morris AJ. Image of the month. Cholesterol embolization. *Gastroenterology.* 2006;130(3):631, 1022.

Giardiello FM, Brensinger JD, Petersen GM. AGA technical review on hereditary colorectal cancer and genetic testing. Gastroenterology. 2001;121(1):198-213.

Gisbert JP, Gonzalez-Lama Y, Mate J. Thiopurine-induced liver injury in patients with inflammatory bowel disease: a systematic review. *Am J Gastroenterol.* 2007;102(7):1518-1527.

Green MH, Duell RM, Johnson CD, Jamieson NV. Haemobilia. *Br J Surg.* 2001;88(6):773-786.

Green PH, Cellier C. Celiac disease. *N Engl J Med.* 2007;357(17):1731-1743.

Green RM, Flamm S. AGA technical review on the evaluation of liver chemistry tests. *Gastroenterology.* 2002;123(4):1367-1384.

Gustafson S, Zbuk KM, Scacheri C, Eng C. Cowden syndrome. *Semin Oncol.* 2007;34(5):428-434.

Hamer DH, Gorbach SL. Infectious diarrhea and bacterial food poisoning. In: Feldman M, Friedman LS, Sleisenger MH, eds. *Sleisenger & Fordtran's Gastrointestinal and Liver Disease: Pathophysiology/Diagnosis/Management.* Vol 2. 7th ed. Philadelphia: Saunders; 2002:1864-1913.

Harish K, Gokulan C. Selective amyloidosis of the small intestine presenting as malabsorption syndrome. *Trop Gastroenterol.* 2008;29(1):37-39.

Helmy A. Review article: updates in the pathogenesis and therapy of hepatic sinusoidal obstruction syndrome. *Aliment Pharmacol Ther.* 2006;23(1):11-25.

Hwang JH, Rulyak SD, Kimmey MB; American Gastroenterological Association Institute technical review on the management of gastric subepithelial masses. *Gastroenterology.* 2006;130(7):2217-2228.

Joyce A, Long WB. Gallstones and gallbladder disorders. In: Ginsberg GG, Ahmad NA, ed. *The Clinician's Guide to Pancreaticobiliary Disorders.* Thorofare, NJ: SLACK Incorporated; 2006;21-45.

Krauss N, Schuppan D. Monitoring nonresponsive patients who have celiac disease. *Gastrointest Endosc Clin N Am.* 2006;16(2):317-327.

Laine L. Mangement of acute colonic pseudoobstruction. *N Engl J Med.* 1999;341(3):192-193.

Lee CC, Lee CW. Clinical challenges and images in GI. Epiploic appendagitis. *Gastroenterology.* 2008;134(7):1829, 2196.

Lee KF, Wong J, Li JC, Lai PB. Polypoid lesions of the gallbladder. *Am J Surg.* 2004;188(2):186-190.

Lew EA, Poles MA, Dieterich DT. Diarrheal diseases associated with HIV infection. *Gastroenterol Clin North Am.* 1997;26(2):259-290.

Levine MS, Buck JL, Pantongrag-Brown L, Buetow PC, Hallman JR, Sobin LH. Fibrovascular polyps of the esophagus: clinical, radiographic, and pathologic findings in 16 patients. *AJR Am J Roentgenol.* 1996;166(4):781-787.

Lindley KJ, Andrews PL. Pathogenesis and treatment of cyclical vomiting. *J Pediatr Gastroenterol Nutr.* 2005;41: S38-40.

Luthen R, Janzik U, Derichs R, Ballo H, Ramp U. Giant fibrovascular polyp of the esophagus. *Eur J Gastroenterol Hepatol.* 2006;18(9):1005-1009.

Madisch A, Miehlke S, Neuber F, et al. Healing of lymphocytic gastritis after Helicobacter pylori eradication therapy—a randomized, double-blind, placebo-controlled multicentre trial. *Aliment Pharmacol Ther.* 2006;23:473-479.

Metcalfe MS, Wemyss-Holden SA, Maddern GJ. Management dilemmas with choledochal cysts. *Arch Surg.* 2003;138(3):333-339.

Morgan J, Bornstein SL, Karpati AM, et al. Outbreak of leptospirosis among triathlon participants and community residents in Springfield, Illinois, 1998. *Clin Infect Dis.* 2002;34(12):1593-1599.

Nazareno J, Ponich T, Gregor J. Long-term follow-up of trigger point injections for abdominal wall pain. *Can J Gastroenterol.* 2005;19(9):561-565.

Nash S, Marconi S, Sikorska K, Naeem R, Nash G. Role of liver bipsy in the diagosis of hepatic iron overload in the era of genetic testing. *Am J Clin Pathol.* 2002;118(1):73-81.

Nielsen OH, Vainer B, Rask-Madsen J. Non-IBD and noninfectious colitis. *Nat Clin Pract Gastroenterol Hepatol.* 2008;5(1):28-39.

No Author. Case records of the Massachusetts General Hospital. Weekly clinicopathological exercises. Case 22-2001. A 25-year-old woman with fever and abnormal liver function. *N Engl J Med.* 2001;345(3):201-205.

Ozturk R, Niazi S, Stessman M, Rao SS. Long-term outcome and objective changes of anorectal function after biofeedback therapy for faecal incontinence. *Aliment Pharmacol Ther.* 2004;20(6):667-674.

Pandolfino JE, Kahrilas PJ. AGA technical review on the clinical use of esophageal manometry. *Gastroenterology.* 2005;128(1):209-224.

Parikh S, Hyman D. Hepatocellular cancer: a guide for the internist. *Am J Med.* 2007;120(3):194-202.

Perlmutter DH. Alpha-1-antitrypsin deficiency. *Clin Liv Dis.* 2000;4(2):220-229.

Petre S, Shah IA, Gilani N. Review article: gastrointestinal amyloidosis-clinical features, diagnosis and therapy. *Aliment Pharmacol Ther.* 2008 ;27(11):1006-1016.

Remorgida V, Ferrero S, Fulcheri E, Ragni N, Martin DC. Bowel endometriosis: presentation, diagnosis, and treatment. *Obstet Gynecol Surv.* 2007;62(7):461-470.

Regev A. Benign and malignant tumors of the liver. In: Reddy K, Faust T, eds. *The Clinician's Guide to Liver Disease.* Thorofare, NJ: SLACK Incorporated; 2006:187-209.

Romagnuolo J, Sadowski DC, Lalor E, Jewell L, Thomson AB. Cholestatic hepatocellular injury with azathioprine: a case report and review of the mechanisms of hepatotoxicity. *Can J Gastroenterol.* 1998;12(7):479-483.

Runyon BA; Practice Guidelines Committee, American Association for the Study of Liver Diseases (AASLD). Management of adult patients with ascites due to cirrhosis. *Hepatology.* 2004;39(3):841-856.

Sandhu BS, Sanyal AJ. Pregnancy and liver disease. *Gastroenterol Clin N Am.* 2003;32(1):407-436.

Schubert ML, Peura DA. Control of gastric acid secretion in health and disease. *Gastroenterology.* 2008;134(7):1842-1860.

Simon A, van der Meer JW, Drenth JP. Familial Mediterranean fever—a not so unusual cause of abdominal pain. *Best Pract Res Clin Gastroenterol.* 2005;19(2):199-213.

Spechler SJ. AGA technical review on treatment of patients with dysphagia caused by benign disorders of the distal esophagus. *Gastroenterology.* 1999;117(1):233-254.

Talley NJ, Vakil N. Practice Parameters Committee of the American College of Gastroenterology. Guidelines for the management of dyspepsia. *Am J Gastroenterol.* 2005;100(10):2324-2337.

Tang RS, Weinberg B, Dawson DW, et al. Evaluation of the guidelines for management of pancreatic branch-duct intraductal papillary mucinous neoplasm. *Clin Gastroenterol Hepatol.* 2008;6(7):815-819.

Tavill AS. Diagnosis and management of hemochromatosis. AASLD Practice Guidelines. *Hepatology.* 2001; 33(5): 1321-1328.

Temino VM, Peebles RS. The spectrum and treatment of angioedema. *Am J Med.* 2008;121(4):282-286.

Thom K, Forrest G. Gastrointestinal infections in immunocompromised hosts. *Curr Opin Gastroenterol.* 2006;22(1):18-23.

Vila N, Millan M, Ferrer X, Riutort N, Escudero D. Levels of alpha1-antitrypsin in plasma and risk of spontaneous cervical artery dissections: a case-control study. *Stroke.* 2003;34(9):E168-169.

Ward EM, Wolfsen HC. Review article: the non-inherited gastrointestinal polyposis syndromes. Aliment Pharmacol Ther. 2002;16(3):333-342.

Ward SK, Roenigk HH, Gordon KB. Dermatological manifestations of gastrointestinal disorders. *Gastrointest Clin North Am.* 1998;27(3):615-636.

Weyant MJ, Maluccio MA, Bertagnolli MM, Daly JM. Choledochal cysts in adults: a report of 2 cases and review of the literature. *Am J Gastroenterol.* 1998;93(12):2580-2583.

Wilcox CM, Rabeneck L, Friedman S. AGA technical review: malnutrition and cachexia, chronic diarrhea, and hepatobiliary disease in patients with human immunodeficiency virus infection. *Gastroenterology.* 1996;111(6):1724-1752.

Wilcox CM, Saag MS. Gastrointestinal complications of HIV infection: changing priorities in the HAART era. *Gut.* 2008;57(6):861-870.

Yonem O, Bayraktar Y. Secondary amyloidosis due to FMF. *Hepatogastroenterology.* 2007;54(76):1061-1065.

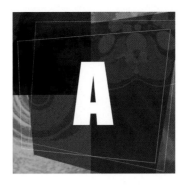

APPENDIX A:
ANSWERS TO "CRUNCH-TIME"
SELF TEST

1. Cowden's syndrome

2. Methhemoglobinemia

3. Renal cell carcinoma

4. Carcinoid syndrome

5. Pyoderma gangrenosum

6. Norwalk virus

7. Glucagonoma

8. Plasmacytoma (with underlying multiple myeloma)

9. Tropical sprue

10. Pseudoxanthoma elasticum (PXE)

11. Acute mesenteric infarction

12. Crycopharyngeus "bar"

13. Gastrointestinal Stromal Tumor (GIST)

14. Median arcuate ligament syndrome

15. Oxalate stone

16. Main branch intraductal papillary mucosal tumor (IPMN)

17. Whipple's disease

18. *Mycobacterium avium intracellulare* (MAC)

19. Herpes simplex virus (HSV) proctitis

20. *Entomoeba histolytica*

21. *Cytomegalovirus* (CMV) colitis

22. Melkersson-Rosenthal Syndrome (Orofacial Crohn's)

23. Leiomyoma

24. Epiploic appendigitis

25. Gastrointestinal amyloidosis

26. Small intestinal bacterial overgrowth (SIBO)

27. Menetrier's Disease

28. Hemosiderosis from iron overload

29. Splenic vein thrombosis

30. Veno-occlusive disease (VOD) or Sinusoidal Obstructive Syndrome (SOS)

31. Dyssynergic defecation

32. Cronkhite-Canada Syndrome

33. Fibrovascular polyp of esophagus

34. Fundic gland polyposis

35. Alpha-1 antitrypsin deficiency

36. Celiac sprue

37. Multiple endocrine neoplasia (MEN) type I (Werner's Syndrome)

38. Sphincter of Oddi Dysfunction (SOD) type I

39. Viral hepatitis

40. Cholesterol embolization to colon

41. Boerhaave'e Syndrome

42. Antral predominant *H. pylori* infection

43. Cronkhite-Canada Syndrome (I had to put this one in twice!)

44. Cryptosporidiosis with terminal ileal involvement

45. Menetrier's Disease

46. Gastric cancer with acanthosis nigricans

47. Non-neutrocytic bacterascites (NNBA)

48. Hereditary angioedema

49. Tylosis (Howell Evans Syndrome)

50. Peliosis Hepatis (*Bartonella henslae*)

51. Lymphocytic gastritis

52. Aortoenteric fistula

53. Hemobilia

54. GI endometriosis

55. Typhlitis

56. Choledochocele (Type III choledochal cyst)

57. Zinc deficiency

58. Schistosomiasis

59. MEN-I with small bowel carcinoid

60. Retained antrum syndrome

61. Blue Rubber Bleb Nevus Syndrome

62. Hemosuccus pancreaticus

63. Temporal arteritis

64. Pancreatic sarcoidosis

65. Listeriosis

66. *Bacillus cerus*

67. Enterohemorrhagic *E. coli*

68. *Vibrio parahemolyticus* or *Vibrio vulnificus*

69. Low levels of TPMT

70. Carbohydrate malabsorption

71. Glomus tumor

72. Schwanomma

73. Duplication cyst

74. Alpha-1 antitrypsin deficiency

75. Paraneoplastic achalasia from lung cancer

76. Combined variable immunodeficiency (CVID)

77. Autoimmune hepatitis

78. Bile salt deficiency with fat malabsorption

79. Acute fatty liver of pregnancy (AFLP)

80. Pancreaticopleural fistula

81. Hereditary nonpolyposis colorectal cancer (HNPCC)

82. Systemic sclerosis

83. Chagas disease

84. Autoimmune pancreatitis

85. Myofascial abdominal wall pain

86. Pyridoxine (vitamin B6) deficiency

87. Niacin deficiency

88. Molybdenum deficiency

89. Immunoproliferative small intestinal disease (IPSID)

90. Selenium deficiency

91. Celiac sprue with dermatitis herpetiformis

92. Familial Mediterranean Fever (FMF)

93. *Entomoeba histolytica*

94. VIPoma

95. Porphyria

96. Cryoglobulinemia

97. Neurofibromatosis

98. Adult Hirschprung's disease

99. *E. coli* 0157:H7 with HUS-TTP

100. Paget's disease

101. Wilson's disease

102. Vitamin A overdose

103. Mastocytosis

104. Acalculous cholecystitis

105. Henoch-Schonlein purpura

106. Churg-Strauss syndrome

107. Somatostatinoma

108. Pill esophagitis with erosion into atrium

109. Dysphagia lusoria (ie, aberrant right subclavian artery compressing the esophagus)

110. Pernicious anemia

111. Pancreatic head cancer

112. Gallstone ileus

113. Focal Nodular Hyperplasia (FNH)

114. Glucagonoma

115. Esophageal glycogenic acanthosis

116. Ogilve's syndrome

117. von Hippel Lindau disease

118. HCV related lichen planus

119. *Vibrio vulnificus*

120. Colon cancer with sign of Lesser Trelat

121. Inadequate fluconazole absorption from PPI-induced hypochlorhydria

122. Congenital chloridorrhea

123. Cyclical vomiting syndrome (CVS)

124. Type III bile duct cyst (choledochocele)

125. Salmonella

126. Typhoid fever (*Salmonella* typhi)

127. Hepatitis B pre-core mutant

128. Idiopathic esophageal ulcer (IEU)—likely HIV itself

129. Comorbid microscopic colitis (Oher differential=lymphoma, true "refractory sprue")

130. Bile salt diarrhea

131. Hereditary nonpolyposis colorectal cancer (HNPCC)

132. Recurrent pyogenic cholangitis ("Oriental Cholangiohepatitis")

133. Hereditary hemochromatosis

134. Leptospirosis

135. Diversion colitis

136. Abetalipoproteinemia

137. Cholestasis of pregnancy

138. Hidradenitis suppurativa from underlying Crohn's Disease

139. Pneumatosis Cystoides Intestinalis

140. Amyloidosis

141. Annular pancreas

142. Dermatomyositis

143. Neuroleptic Malignant Syndrome from Compazine (prochlorperazine)

144. Proctalgia fugax

145. Hypercalcemia

146. Cardiac angina with radiation to the epigastrium

147. Rheumatoid arthritis

148. Gardner's syndrome

149. Pernicious anemia

150. Felty's syndrome

151. Colon cancer

152. Antibiotic-precipitated HUS-TTP

153. Intestinal lymphangiectasia

154. Thiamine deficiency

155. Gastrointestinal amyloidosis

156. *Isospora belli* enteritis

157. Trousseau's sign and depression from underlying pancreatic cancer
158. Variegated porphyria
159. Plummer-Vinson Syndrome
160. Gastric outlet obstruction
161. Cervical osteophyte
162. Eosinophilic esophagitis
163. Hepatic adenoma
164. Nodular regenerative hyperplasia (NRH) of the liver
165. Carbohydrate malabsorption (eg, lactase deficiency, chewing gum diarrhea)
166. Primary biliary cirrhosis (PBC)
167. Crohn's Disease with gastric involvement
168. Pseudolipomatosis (insufflation artifact)
169. Bechet's Disease
170. Ehlers-Danlos Syndrome

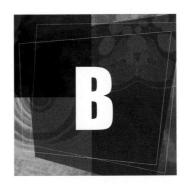

APPENDIX B
"CRUNCH-TIME" SELF TEST
SCORING GUIDE

170 correct: You cheated.

160-169: You still cheated.

150-159: Either you cheated, or you're a monster diagnostician ready to crush the Boards.

140-149: Assuming you didn't cheat, that was a crazy good performance.

130-139: Outstanding performance—easily a standard deviation above the mean.

120-129: Highly respectable—well above average for this level of difficulty.

110-119: Good work—you're ahead of the curve.

100-109: Don't despair—these are hard, and you hung in well.

90-99: Not terrible, but you need to fine tune the rough spots.

80-89: You're in the 50% correct range now—not awesome.

70-79: Sub-par but not a total disaster. You need to go back and study.

60-69: Not good enough—below average.

50-59: These are tough, but you're well below the curve.

40-49: Inadequate knowledge base. You're in jeopardy of not passing the exam.

<39: Wait a while before taking the exam. You've got a ways to go.

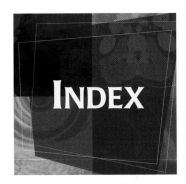

INDEX